AF251995

EUROPEAN SCHOOL OF ONCOLOGY SCIENTIFIC UPDATES, VOLUME 4

Primary Medical Therapy for Breast Cancer: Clinical and Biological Aspects

Primary Medical Therapy for Breast Cancer: Clinical and Biological Aspects

Edited by

Anthony Howell

CRC Department of Medical Oncology
Christie Hospital NHS Trust
Manchester, United Kingdom

Mitch Dowsett

Academic Department of Biochemistry
The Royal Marsden Hospital
London, United Kingdom

1999

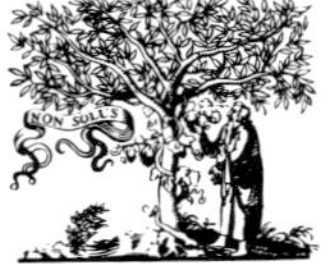

ELSEVIER

AMSTERDAM - LAUSANNE - NEW YORK - OXFORD - SHANNON- SINGAPORE - TOKYO

ELSEVIER SCIENCE B.V.
Sara Burgerhartstraat 25
P.O. Box 211, 1000 AE Amsterdam, The Netherlands

First edition 1999

Library of Congress Cataloging in Publication Data
A catalog record from the Library of Congress has been applied for.

ISBN: 0 444 50327 7

The European School of Oncology gratefully acknowledges
sponsorship for the production of this book from an
unrestricted educational grant from

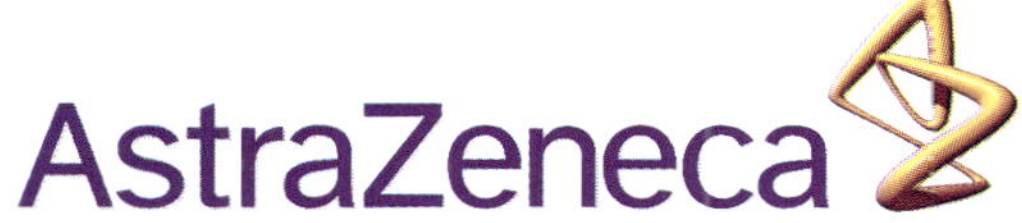

Foreword

The European School of Oncology (ESO) is a non-governmental, non profit-making organisation, which was founded in 1982. It has since become a model for many other professional groups that need to provide timely information, education and training. The rate of progress in the areas of diagnosis and treatment of cancer is so rapid that oncologists need continuous updating in order to provide their patients the best chances for palliation or cure. ESO recognises the multidisciplinary nature of cancer treatment, and its activities encompass all medical, nursing and technical specialities dealing with neoplastic diseases. Timeliness and scientific accuracy are the key factors behind the numerous activities of the School.

One of the many initiatives of ESO has been the institution of study groups, also called task forces, where leading experts exchange views on the state of the art of a given field, discuss controversies and new developments, and give opinions on future directions. These groups often publish a summary in a peer-reviewed journal, or excerpts of the discussions are presented as "Newsletters". The *Scientific Updates* are a series of books designed to disseminate the full results of such discussions. Each issue is under the responsibility of one or several volume editors, and contains the latest information on a particular topic.

To preserve the timeliness of the information, the ESO *Scientific Updates* utilise a simple layout and presentation to enable very rapid publication times, thus overcoming a common problem in the medical literature: that of the material being outdated even before publication.

The editors welcome suggestions for further issues and, together with the whole ESO staff, are ready to help interested parties in establishing new task force meetings. In this way the knowledge of new developments in all fields of oncology, from research through to nursing, can be shared. Education and training are important in helping reduce cancer-related mortality, and the ESO is firmly committed to achieving this aim.

Matti S. Aapro
ESO Scientific Updates
Series Editor

Umberto Veronesi
Chairman Scientific Committee
European School of Oncology

Contents

ESO Scientific Updates, Vol. 4
Primary Medical Therapy for Breast Cancer
A. Howell and M. Dowsett, editors
© 1999 Elsevier Science B.V. All rights reserved

Introduction

Anthony Howell and Mitch Dowsett

The Breast Cancer Task Force of the European School of Oncology met at Runnymede, near London, in January 1999. The aim of this session was to review the clinical and biological data related to the use of primary medical therapy (PMT) in breast cancer. A large number of primary endocrine and chemotherapy trials have been performed together with several associated laboratory studies. PMT has been with us for over 20 years now, so it was thought to be of value to bring together many of the leading investigators in the area. This allowed us to produce a summary of the current status of PMT, as outlined in this volume, and to discuss new approaches which are required to progress PMT in breast cancer patients.

Primary endocrine therapy, usually consisting of tamoxifen, was initially given in phase II studies to determine whether it was possible to avoid surgery in elderly women presenting with primary breast tumours. The four randomised trials comparing surgery with tamoxifen were undertaken to test the safety of delaying surgery. Primary chemotherapy was initially used to treat locally advanced and inflammatory tumours and later to assess its effectiveness in downstaging tumours to allow more frequent breast conservation surgery. Numerous phase II trials indicated that this was feasible and led to five phase III trials where the aim was to determine whether primary chemotherapy produced a survival advantage compared with adjuvant chemotherapy.

More recently new endocrine and chemotherapies have been assessed for their applicability as primary treatments. For example, high and rapid response rates were seen by the Edinburgh Group using preoperative third-generation aromatase inhibitors (letrozole and anastrozole), which may be superior to the commonly used tamoxifen. For chemotherapy high response rates to infusional chemotherapy, dose-intensified treatments and taxanes have been reported.

The primary tumour provides an ideal scenario for assessing predictive biomarkers and hypothetical molecular relationships in that it allows measurements to be made before, during and after treatment and for these measurements to be related to clinical outcome. To date, markers of proliferation, cell death, drug resistance and metastases have been studied by a variety of techniques in order to predict tumour behaviour and patient outcome. At present, few markers have entered routine use but the advent of new, high-throughput techniques may change this situation soon.

The meeting has resulted in this publication, the fourth volume in the ESO Scientific Update series, which we hope will be a useful summary for those who work or wish to work in this increasingly productive area of breast cancer investigation.

In the section on the study of biomarkers reference is made to many genes and their products. There are internationally accepted guidelines on the nomenclature to be used, but in this book (as in the majority of other publications) authors have not universally adhered to this convention. We do not believe that there is a risk of misinterpretation.

We would like to thank all the contributors to the meeting and to this review, the European School of Oncology for organising the meeting, and the sponsor for the generous financial support. Finally, without the persistence and talented help of Marije de Jager it would not have been possible to produce this timely report.

ESO Scientific Updates, Vol. 4
Primary Medical Therapy for Breast Cancer
A. Howell and M. Dowsett, editors

Primary Medical Treatment: The Results of the NSABP-B18 Trial and the Royal Marsden Hospital Trial

Laura Assersohn and Trevor J. Powles

Breast Unit, Royal Marsden Hospital (London and Surrey), Downs Road, Sutton, Surrey SM2 5PT, United Kingdom

Introduction

Clinical trials have clearly shown that the use of adjuvant chemotherapy after surgical treatment for primary breast cancer will improve the control of local and systemic disease. In addition, experimental studies have indicated that animals treated with chemotherapy or tamoxifen prior to surgery have improved survival. This could possibly result from a reduction in surgical dissemination or from a reduction in circulating growth factors, inhibited by chemotherapy, prior to surgery. This raises the possibility that use of chemotherapy before surgery (neoadjuvant therapy) could be more effective than after surgery for treatment of primary operable breast cancer. Various randomised trials have been undertaken, the largest of which is the NSABP-B18 trial [1,2]. The Royal Marsden Hospital is a smaller but comparable trial which had similar objectives for the evaluation of primary medical treatment in stage I and II breast cancer [3].

The primary aim of these trials was to assess whether chemotherapy given in the neoadjuvant setting would have superior efficacy in terms of disease-free survival (DFS) and overall survival (OS) compared with the same treatment given in the adjuvant setting. These studies were also designed to determine whether the administration of chemotherapy prior to surgery would decrease the requirements for mastectomy and influence the local relapse rate.

Pathological studies in these trials could show whether there was also downstaging in the axillary nodes caused by the treatment. Another objective of the trials was to test whether the response in the primary tumour to neoadjuvant treatment would correlate with disease-free survival and overall survival and thereby be a marker of the response of micrometastases to chemotherapy.

Address for correspondence: T.J. Powles, Breast Unit, Royal Marsden Hospital, Downs Road, Sutton, Surrey SM2 5PT, United Kingdom. Tel.: +44-181-6613361, fax: +44-181-7707313, e-mail trevor.powles@rmh.nthames.nhs.uk

Women with primary operable breast cancer were recruited to both trials. In the NSABP-B18 trial, four courses of adriamycin (60 mg/m^2) and cyclophosphamide (600 mg/m^2) (AC) were given every three weeks either prior to surgery (neoadjuvant) or after surgery (adjuvant). In the RMH trial mitoxantrone (11 mg/m^2) and methotrexate (35 mg/m^2) (MM) with or without mitomycin C (MMM) were given every three weeks. In the adjuvant group eight courses of MM(M) were given after surgery, whilst in the neoadjuvant group four courses of MM(M) were given prior to surgery and four courses after surgery. Thus, in the RMH trial all patients who had conservation surgery received chemotherapy concurrently with postoperative radiotherapy, including a boost to the tumour bed, contrary to the NSABP-B18 trial which administered only four courses of chemotherapy before or after surgery and not at the time of radiotherapy and with no boost given to the tumour bed. In the RMH trial all patients received tamoxifen 20 mg/day whilst only women aged over 50 received tamoxifen in the NSABP-B18 trial. Tamoxifen was given in both studies regardless of oestrogen and progesterone receptor status.

NSABP-B18 trial

Fifteen hundred women were randomised to adjuvant or neoadjuvant AC chemotherapy in this multicentre trial between October 1988 and April 1993. Patients were well balanced between the two treatment groups for age, menopausal status, clinical tumour size and clinical nodal status. At the time of randomisation approximately 50% of patients were premenopausal and 30% of patients had relatively small T1 primary cancers.

The response rate to AC chemotherapy for patients randomised to neoadjuvant therapy was high. Two hundred and forty-eight patients (36%) achieved a clinical complete response (cCR), 43% had a clinical partial response (PR) while 20% had stable or progressive disease. Histological examination of the surgical samples from patients who achieved cCR showed that 89 patients (13% of the total neoadjuvant group) had a pathological complete response (pCR) (Table 1). The pathological nodal status was examined for patients according to their response. Of the patients who achieved a pCR, 87% had no evidence of axillary node involvement at the time of surgery, compared with 62% of cCR patients, 56% of PR patients and 47% of non-responders.

The very high objective response rate was associated with reduced requirements for mastectomy. Of the 487 patients who were randomised to neoadjuvant chemotherapy, 256 (34.5%) were considered to require mastectomy but after chemotherapy, with associated response, only 187 patients (25%) actually required mastectomy. There was a downstaging in the clinical node status of the patients with 185 (25%) having clinical evidence of axillary lymph node involvement before chemotherapy and only 50 (7%) after chemotherapy (Table 2).

Table 1. Primary breast cancer response to neoadjuvant chemotherapy

	NSABP-B18 (683)			RMH (144)		
pCR	89*	(13%)		19**	(13%)	
cCR	248	(36%)		32	(22%)	
MRD	–	–	79%	9	(29%)	84%
PR	295	(43%)		47	(33%)	
NC/PD	140	(20%)		24	(16%)	

* only evaluated in cCR
** includes 9 residual DCIS only

Table 2. Surgical requirements, T stage and clinical lymph node status in 743 patients receiving neoadjuvant adriamycin and cyclophosphamide in NSABP-B18 and 149 patients receiving neoadjuvant mitoxantrone and methotrexate (mitomycin C) in the RMH trial

	NSABP (743)				RMH (149)			
	Pre-chemo		Post-chemo		Pre-chemo		Post-chemo	
Lumpectomy	487		435		114		132	
Mastectomy	256	(34.5%)	187	(25%)	35	(23.5%)	16	(10.7%)*
Clinical N0	558		693		117		145	
Clinical N1	185	(25%)	50	(7%)	32	(21.5%)	4	(2.7%)**
T 0-1	215	(29%)	–		16	(10%)	118	(79%)**
T2	431	(58%)	–		129		28	
T3	97	(13%)	–		4		1	

* $p = 0.004$
** $p = 0.0001$

After a median follow-up of five years there were no differences in disease-free ($p = 0.99$) or overall ($p = 0.83$) survival for the patients who received adjuvant or neoadjuvant chemotherapy [2]. There was also no significant difference in the incidence of regional or distant relapse rates for the two groups (Table 3).

Table 3. Local and regional relapse in NSABP-B18 and RMH trial

	NSABP-B18		RMH	
	ADJ (752)	NEOADJ (743)	ADJ (144)	NEOADJ (149)
Distant relapse	126 (16.8%)	120 (16.2%)	28 (19%)	28 (19%)
Regional relapse	24 (3.2%)	22 (3.0%)	5 (3.5%)	4 (2.7%)
Local relapse total	44 (5.8%)	40 (7.9%)		
Proposed and had lumpectomy (435)	–	30 (6.9%)	–	–
Proposed mastectomy; had lumpectomy (69)	–	10 (14.5%)*	–	–

* p = 0.04

The local relapse rate was not significantly (p = 0.22) higher in the neoadjuvant (7.9%) compared to the adjuvant arm (5.8%). There was, however, an indication that patients who were considered to require mastectomy before chemotherapy but were suitable subsequently for lumpectomy (69 patients) had a higher local relapse rate. Only 6.9% of the patients who initially had a lumpectomy proposed, and who subsequently had a lumpectomy, had a local relapse, compared with 14.5% of those who should have had a mastectomy but who, after downstaging, had a lumpectomy (p = 0.04) (Table 3).

Although there was no detectable difference in relapse-free and overall survival between the adjuvant and neoadjuvant groups, there was clearly a difference in survival for patients in the neoadjuvant group who achieved a response versus those who did not. Those patients who achieved a cCR had a significantly increased disease-free survival (p = 0.0014), although at present this is not yet apparent for overall survival (p = 0.19). Those patients who achieved a pCR in response to neoadjuvant chemotherapy had a significantly increased disease-free survival (p = 0.0001). The overall survival for the pCR group is marginally significantly better than for others at this time (p = 0.06), with a decreased relative risk (RR = 0.55, 95% CI, 0.33-0.91) (Fig. 1).

On multivariate analysis the breast tumour response to neoadjuvant chemotherapy was a significant predictor of disease-free survival (p = 0.056), along with pathological nodal status after chemotherapy (p<0.0001) and clinical tumour size at randomisation (p = 0.0005).

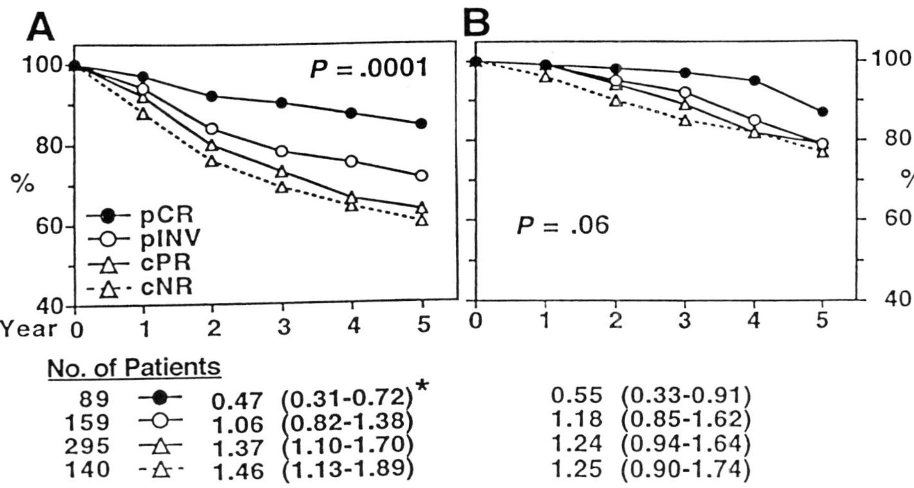

Fig. 1. Effect of preoperative chemotherapy on the outcome of women with operable breast cancer. (A) Disease-free survival; (B) overall survival. * Relative risk (95% CI). pCR, pathological complete response; pINV, invasive cells on pathological examination; cPR, clinical partial response; cNR, no response. Reproduced with permission from [2].

RMH trial

A total of 300 patients were randomised in the RMH single-centre study to receive adjuvant or neoadjuvant MM(M) chemotherapy and tamoxifen (T) between February 1990 and August 1995. Patients were well balanced between the two treatment groups. Approximately 33% of patients were premenopausal, 10% of tumours were T1 and 80% were T2, and 80% of patients had no clinical evidence of axillary node involvement at the time of randomisation. Patients were assessed for clinical response according to the International Union against Cancer Criteria (UICC). However, patients who had a residual palpable abnormality but no palpable measurable lump were classified as minimal residual disease (MRD) and the category of complete clinical response (cCR) and MRD were considered as a group of good clinical response (GCR).

Of the 144 patients who were assessable for clinical response to neoadjuvant MM(M), 22% achieved a cCR, 29% MRD, 33% a PR and 16% of patients were classified as non-responders (NC/PD). Thirteen percent of the neoadjuvant cohort achieved a pathological complete response (pCR), including nine patients who had residual DCIS only. These results indicate that the response to MM(M)T is almost identical to the response to AC in NSABP-B18 (Table 1).

This high response rate was associated with a significant downstaging. Only 10% of patients had a T0 or T1 tumour (<2 cm) pre-chemotherapy, compared to 79% post-treatment (Table 2). There was also a significant reduction in the clinical detection of involved lymph nodes, with 21.5% of patients having obvious nodes pre-treatment and only 2.7% post-treatment. As a result of this downstaging, the mastectomy requirements were significantly decreased in the neoadjuvant group. Only 11% of patients required mastectomy after chemotherapy compared with 23.5% of patients having a mastectomy proposed initially (p = 0.004). After a median follow-up of four years there was no difference in disease-free survival (p = 0.8) or overall survival (p = 1.0) for the two treatment groups [4]. The distant relapse rate was identical for the two groups (19%) and the local relapse rate was 3.5% for patients randomised to adjuvant treatment compared to 2.7% for patients randomised to neoadjuvant treatment (Table 3). Of the 20 patients who achieved a pCR only one patient has had a locoregional relapse and this was an isolated lymph node in the ipsilateral axilla.

Like NSABP-B18, although there was no difference in survival between patients randomised to adjuvant versus neoadjuvant treatment, there was a significant difference in survival for patients who responded versus those who did not. Those achieving pCR or GCR had a significantly improved disease-free survival (p = 0.02) and overall survival (p = 0.004) compared to patients who only achieved a partial response or had no response.

Furthermore, a phase II trial undertaken at the Royal Marsden Hospital has also demonstrated encouraging response rates [5]. Fifty patients with median tumour diameters of 6 cm (range, 3-12 cm) received continuous infusional 5-fluorouracil (5FU) (200 mg/m^2/day) with epirubicin (50 mg/m^2) intravenous (iv) bolus and cisplatin (60 mg/m^2) iv bolus (ECF) every three weeks for eight courses. Thirty-three patients (66%; 95% confidence interval 53-79%) had a clinical CR and only three patients required mastectomy. A randomised trial comparing ECF and AC is currently underway to confirm whether ECF has a significantly higher response rate than the regimen employed in NSABP-B18.

Conclusions

The NSABP-B18 and RMH trials clearly demonstrate that neoadjuvant chemotherapy does not improve the disease-free or overall survival compared to the same treatment given as adjuvant therapy. It seems unlikely that this will change with longer follow-up. Downstaging of clinical tumour size and clinical nodal status was evident and similar in both trials and this was associated with a similar reduction in the requirement for mastectomy.

However, local relapse rates were higher in the NSABP-B18 trial compared to the RMH trial for both adjuvant and neoadjuvant therapy, although the period of follow-up was marginally longer for the NSABP study. There was no significant difference in local relapse rates between the two treatment groups for either trial. The relatively higher local relapse rate in the NSABP-B18 trial may relate to the use of radiotherapy. In the RMH trial, patients who had conservation also received a radiation boost to the tumour bed which was not given in the NSABP trial. Another factor may relate to the concomitant use of radiation with chemotherapy in the Royal Marsden trial which was not used in the NSABP trial. It is possible that chemotherapy is able to sensitise any residual tumour cells to radiation and thereby reduce the local relapse rate.

In both trials, responders to neoadjuvant chemotherapy have improved disease-free and overall survival compared with non-responders. It may be that chemotherapy response identifies a subgroup of cancers which are inherently less aggressive. Alternatively, response of the primary breast cancer to chemotherapy may be a surrogate marker of the chemotherapy effect on micrometastases. Nevertheless, as a result of the significantly improved disease-free survival seen with the clinical complete responders, and especially the pathological complete responders, the authors of the NSABP-B18 trial recommended that clinical response to neoadjuvant chemotherapy should be used as an intermediate endpoint for assessment of chemotherapy regimens. In this context it is interesting to note that the absolute benefit from adjuvant chemoendocrine therapy in adjuvant trials is about 10% absolute reduction in mortality. This figure is similar to the complete histological response rate reported with neoadjuvant therapy, which makes it likely that both groups of patients are in fact the same group.

Future direction

The presence of the primary tumour while patients are receiving systemic therapy allows the assessment of the response of individual tumours to treatment regimens and this may reflect the benefit on micrometastases. In the future, the use of more intensive chemotherapy regimens, and possibly the use of taxanes, may increase the pathological response rate, which potentially will be translated into increased disease-free and overall survival. At the present time the results are awaited of the NSABP-B27 trial, which involves women with primary operable breast cancer given neoadjuvant AC with or without Taxol (docetaxel). The objective is to improve the pathological complete response rate and evaluate any impact this will have on disease-free and overall survival.

Use of neoadjuvant chemotherapy, along with assessment of clinical response, allows the evaluation of molecular markers, such as indices of apoptosis and proliferation, in the primary tumour before and during early treatment, thus developing predictive markers of response and methods for monitoring response. This could allow us to optimise treatment to individual patients, in order to identify those patients who may not require systemic treatment and thereby prevent widespread overtreatment of those patients who will not gain benefit.

References

1   Fisher B, Brown A, Mamounas E et al. Effect of preoperative chemotherapy on local-regional disease in women with operable breast cancer: findings from National Surgical Adjuvant Breast and Bowel Project B-18. J Clin Oncol 1997; 15: 2483-93
2   Fisher B, Bryant J, Wolmark N et al. Effect of preoperative chemotherapy on the outcome of women with operable breast cancer. J Clin Oncol 1998; 16: 2672-85
3   Powles TJ, Hickish TF, Makris A et al. Randomized trial of chemoendocrine therapy started before or after surgery for treatment of primary breast cancer. J Clin Oncol 1995; 13: 547-52
4   Makris A, Powles T, Ashley S et al. A reduction in the requirements for mastectomy in a randomized trial of neoadjuvant chemoendocrine therapy in primary breast cancer. Ann Oncol 1998; 9: 1179-84
5   Smith IE, Walsh G, Jones A et al. High complete remission rates with primary neoadjuvant infusional chemotherapy for large early breast cancer. J Clin Oncol 1995; 13: 424-9

ESO Scientific Updates, Vol. 4
Primary Medical Therapy for Breast Cancer
A. Howell and M. Dowsett, editors
© 1999 Elsevier Science B.V. All rights reserved

Primary Chemotherapy: The European Experience

Louis Mauriac, Gaëtan MacGrogan, Antoine Avril and Jean-Marie Dilhuydy

Institut Bergonié, Regional Cancer Center, Bordeaux, France

Introduction

Primary chemotherapy has been applied since the 1970s. It has four justifications: historical, theoretical, experimental and clinical. In 1943 Haagensen defined inoperability criteria on the basis of a retrospective analysis of more than 1000 breast cancers: operated breast tumours associated with erythema, "peau d'orange" or cutaneous infiltration had a 5-year local relapse rate of 48% and a metastasis-free survival of only 3% [1]. Given this very low survival rate, it seemed important to use other treatments which would be able to treat micrometastatic disease already present at the diagnostic stage.

In 1959 the usefulness of cyclophosphamide was assessed in rat chloroleukoma: while local treatment alone cured 15% of cases, pretreatment with this drug increased the rate to 28%, and even to 90% when pretreatment was applied earlier. Furthermore, Fisher showed that incomplete surgical excision of a tumour was associated with an increase in residual tumour cells [2]. The doubling time of these cells, assessed by the thymidine labelling index, was seen to rise for a few days following surgery. This phenomenon was due to a growth stimulating factor induced by local treatment [3]. The use of chemotherapy delivered before local surgical treatment would prevent the modifications of cell kinetics and could lessen the aggressiveness of these cells.

An experimental justification is based on the hypothesis of Goldie and Coldman [4,5]: the number of chemoresistant cells is positively correlated with the total number of tumour cells while the number of somatic mutations increases. So, it was thought that it would be possible to lessen these mutations, which are associated with an increased risk of chemoresistance, by delivering non-crossresistant drugs when the tumour volume is as small as possible. The number of chemoresistant cells will decrease, as will the subsequent risk of secondary chemoresistance of cells which would still be chemosensitive.

Address for correspondence: L. Mauriac, Department of Medicine, Institut Bergonié, Regional Cancer Center, 180, rue de Saint-Genès, 33076 Bordeaux Cedex, France. Tel.: +33-5-56 33 32 58, fax: +33-5-56 33 33 85, e-mail: mauriac@bergonie.org

Clinical justifications have long been known. After having noted that adjuvant chemotherapy delivered after surgery or irradiation improved the overall and metastasis-free survival, several teams proposed to reverse the order of treatments by applying chemotherapy before local treatment. The first step of this new strategy was conducted in locally advanced and inflammatory breast carcinomas [6]. The results of many phase II trials were published, showing that survival improved in comparison with that of patients treated with local treatments alone. Although this comparison was made in a retrospective analysis, the improvement seemed good enough to allow systematic use of primary chemotherapy for these bad prognosis tumours [7]. Current studies seek to improve the efficacy of chemotherapeutic regimens by using high-dose chemotherapy [8], more intensive chemotherapy [9], or taxanes. This therapeutic approach might therefore be proposed for those operable breast cancers that have a high recurrence rate because of clinical tumour size or poor prognostic factors such as axillary node involvement or absence of hormone receptiveness.

Many phase II trials have been conducted in Europe: in Belgium [10], France [11-15], Italy [16], and the United Kingdom [17,18]. They did show the feasibility of such a treatment strategy but none of them was able to demonstrate that primary chemotherapy could maintain the benefit obtained by classical adjuvant treatment. It was therefore necessary to demonstrate such a benefit and to show that primary chemotherapy decreased the number of mastectomies which would have been otherwise performed for these large tumours. Four randomised phase III studies have been conducted and published in Europe in eight years: in France [19-21], Russia [22], and the United Kingdom [23]. We will discuss the French and Russian trials here; the latest UK randomised trial was published recently and is discussed elsewhere in this volume [see chapter by Assersohn and Powles].

European randomised phase III studies

Institut Bergonié trial [19, 20]

The trial was conducted from January 1985 to April 1989 and recruited 272 women. All of them had T2 tumours larger than 3 cm on clinical examination or T3 with or without clinical nodal involvement. T4 tumours as well as N2 and N3 tumours were excluded. No metastatic disease was present as assessed by chest X-ray, bone scan and biological liver analysis. Core biopsy was performed to obtain a pathological diagnosis and oestrogen and progesterone receptor (ER/PgR) status was determined by dextran-coated charcoal (DCC) microtitration with a single saturating dose [24].

For pathological examination, samples were processed by Bouin-Hollande fixation, paraffin embedding and haematoxylin-eosin (HES) staining. All included patients had a diagnosis of infiltrating breast carcinoma. The patients' characteristics were identical in the two treatment arms with respect to age,

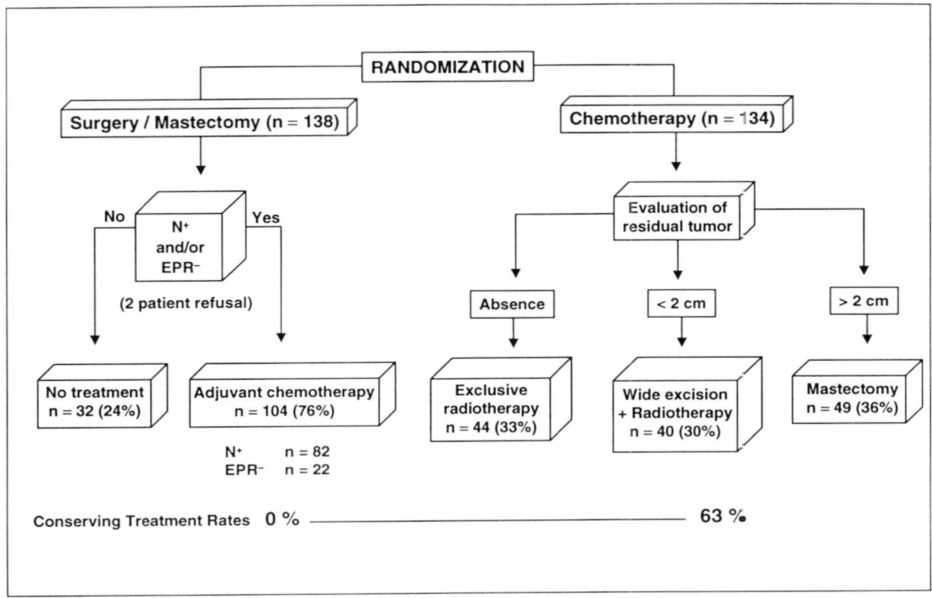

Fig. 1. Treatment schedule of Institut Bergonié trial.

menopausal status, initial tumour size, TNM classification, pathological types, Scarff-Bloom-Richardson (SBR) grading and, for women in the initial surgery group, tumour size and nodal involvement.

After oral informed consent had been obtained from all patients, treatment was chosen by randomisation (Fig. 1). Patients treated with initial surgery (group A, n=138) underwent modified radical mastectomy (MRM) followed by adjuvant chemotherapy in case of pathological nodal involvement or in case of absence of the two receptors (ER/PgR−). The first course was delivered before the 15th day post-mastectomy. Irradiation was not performed in this group.

Patients treated with neoadjuvant chemotherapy (n=134) (group B) received the first treatment course by the fourth day after the core biopsy result. Tumour regression was regularly assessed after the first, third and sixth courses by a multidisciplinary team comprising a surgeon, a radiotherapist and a medical oncologist; the assessment was based on clinical examination and mammography. Locoregional treatment was performed within the following 21 days and depended on tumour regression: irradiation of the breast and nodal areas was performed in case of complete clinical regression; in case of residual tumour smaller than 2 cm, lumpectomy and breast irradiation were performed; in case of residual tumour larger than 2 cm, modified radical mastectomy without irradiation was performed. The irradiation modalities were described in the initial report [19].

Chemotherapy was the same in both treatment groups. Six courses were delivered, one every three weeks. The first three courses consisted of epirubicin (50 mg/m^2), vincristine (1 mg/m^2) and methotrexate (20 mg/m^2), and the last three of mitomycin C (10 mg/m^2), thiotepa (20 mg/m^2) and vindesine (4 mg/m^2). Dose reductions were applied according to haematological toxicity [19]. Because there is no proven improvement in survival by reinforcement or prolongation of adjuvant chemotherapy [25], group B patients who had pathological axillary node involvement received no further neoadjuvant chemotherapy.

We used the log rank test to compare differences between survival curves. Cox's regression analysis was used for survival analysis [26] to determine the influence of different prognostic factors. A difference was considered statistically significant if the p value was less than 0.05.

The results concern initial response rates, breast conservation rates with long follow-up, and recurrence according to local treatment in group B. In group A all patients had a MRM and 76% received adjuvant chemotherapy (n=104); the others (n=32) did not receive any adjuvant treatment because of the absence of axillary node involvement or steroid receptors. At the date of trial initiation, large tumour size alone was not considered a sufficiently poor prognostic factor to initiate adjuvant chemotherapy or hormone therapy. In group B (n=134) breast conserving surgery after neoadjuvant chemotherapy was performed in 63.1%: 33% (n=44) underwent only irradiation, 30% (n=40) had breast conserving surgery plus breast irradiation, and 36.9% (n=49) had a mastectomy (Fig. 1). At the last analysis (June 1997) the median follow-up was 124 months (range 47-148 months) [20]. When the first sites of relapse were examined, locoregional recurrences proved to be more frequent in group B (n=31) than in group A (n=12), and this was due to breast conservation.

When locoregional relapse occurred general restaging was performed. In cases of metastatic disease associated with locoregional recurrence, medical treatment was applied without salvage mastectomy. Salvage mastectomy was only performed in patients with isolated local and/or regional recurrences.

When the breast conserving treatment rates were analysed according to the ER/PgR status of the primary tumour, initial breast conservation rates were more frequent for ER/PgR-negative tumours (77%) than for ER/PgR-positive tumours (52%). This difference remains constant with time and recurrence is as frequent in ER/PgR-negative tumours as in ER/PgR-positive tumours (Fig. 2).

We studied the number of relapses according to local treatment performed in group B. The number of nodal relapses in patients treated with irradiation alone was higher than that of patients treated with axillary dissection (10 versus 1), but only one of the nodal relapses in the axilla was symptomatic; in two cases the nodal relapse was associated with metastatic disease and the other seven, asymptomatic, nodes were diagnosed after salvage mastectomy with axillary clearance. In patients treated with irradiation alone 15 local relapses were observed: six were isolated in the breast, seven were associated with axillary nodal involvement and two with axillary nodal involvement and metastasis. In patients treated with lumpectomy nine local relapses were ob-

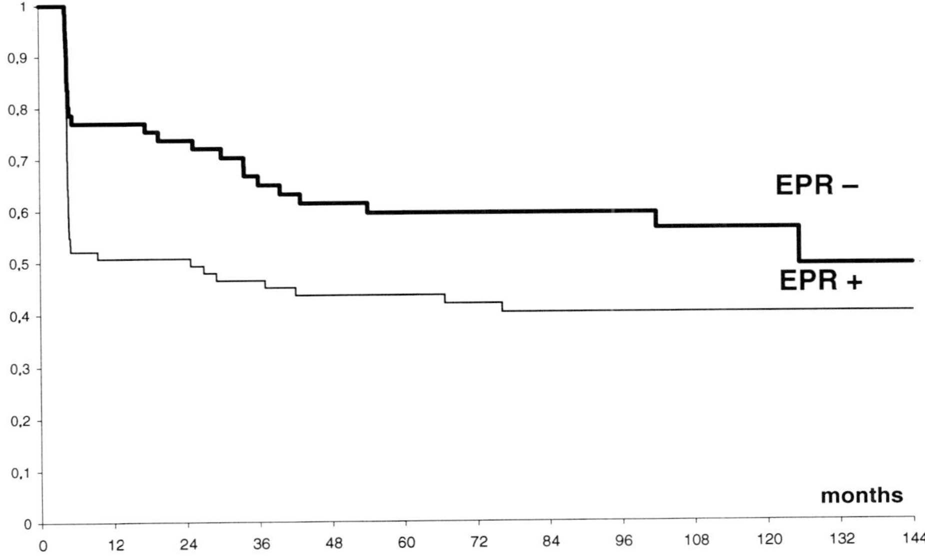

Fig. 2. Breast conserving treatment curves according to ER/PgR status in group B.

served: six were isolated in the breast and three were locoregional recurrences with metastasis. In patients treated with MRM 11 locoregional relapses were observed: seven in the scar, one was associated with axillary node recurrence and the remaining three were associated with metastasis (Table 1).

Table 1. Institut Bergonié trial. Relapses according to local treatment in the preoperative chemotherapy group

	Only irradiation to breast and nodal areas	Lumpectomy + axillary dissection + breast irradiation	Mastectomy + axillary dissection without irradiation
Patients (n)	44	40	49
Relapses (n)	21	17	28
Local	15	9	11
breast	6	6	–
breast + axilla	7	–	–
breast + axilla + metastasis	2	–	–
breast + metastasis	–	3	–
Nodal	10	–	1
Metastasis	7	11	20

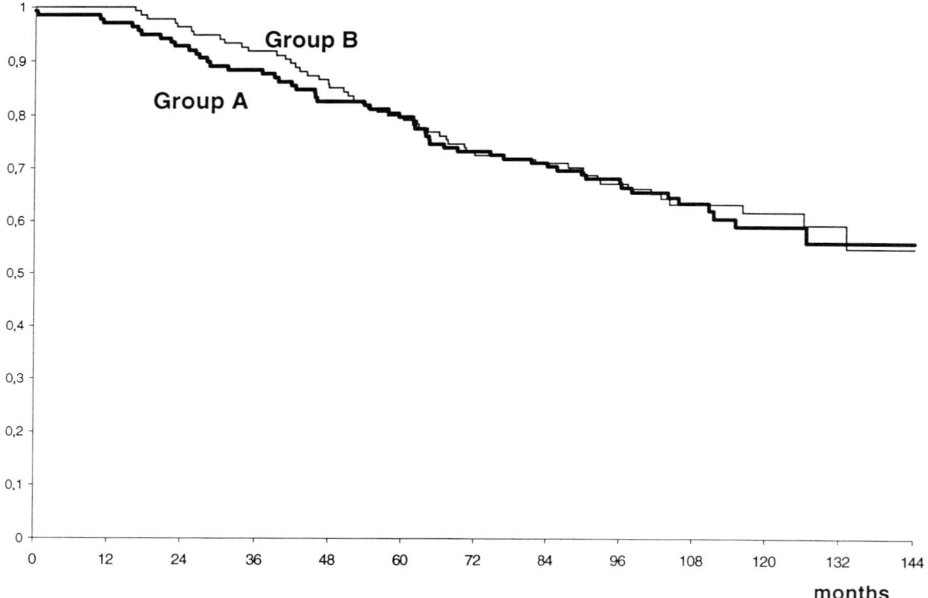

Fig. 3. Overall survival of patients treated with primary surgery (group A) or primary chemotherapy (group B).

At the first analysis in 1991 with a 34-month median follow-up, the recurrence-free survival of all patients of groups A and B was equivalent whereas the overall survival was better for group B patients treated with neoadjuvant chemotherapy [19] (Fig. 3). This difference disappeared with a longer follow-up, and at present the overall survival, metastasis-free survival and recurrence-free survival are identical (curves not shown) [20].

Institut Curie trial [21]

This trial also analysed the potential advantage in survival with primary chemotherapy as compared to adjuvant chemotherapy in premenopausal women with operable T2-T3 N0-N1 M0 breast cancer. Treatment was randomised between primary chemotherapy followed by adapted locoregional treatment or primary locoregional treatment (irradiation followed or not by surgery) and adjuvant chemotherapy (Fig. 4). In the primary chemotherapy group, tumour regression was assessed after two courses and chemotherapy was continued up to four courses if tumour shrinkage was observed. If there was no tumour regression, local treatment was performed. In the other treatment arm surgical removal of residual tumour after breast irradiation was performed and aimed to be as conservative as possible. Adjuvant chemotherapy was given afterwards to patients with poor prognostic factors. The chemotherapy regimen, whether deliv-

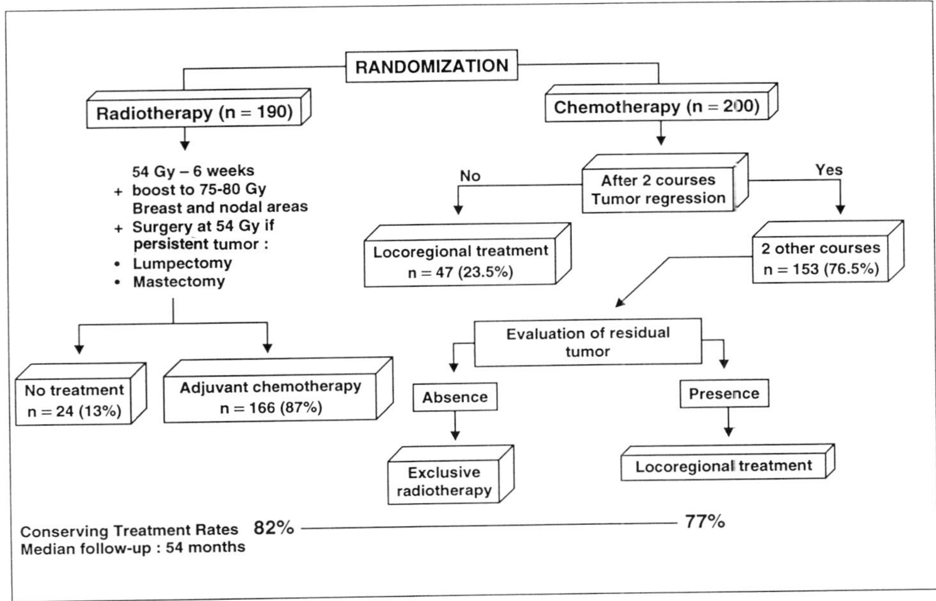

Fig. 4. Treatment schedule of Institut Curie trial.

ered as primary or as adjuvant treatment, consisted of cyclophosphamide 500 mg/m^2 on day 1 and day 8, doxorubicin 25 mg/m^2 on day 1 and day 8 and 5FU 500 mg/m^2 on days 1, 3 and 5. Among the 414 patients enrolled, 390 were evaluable. At the time of publication of the first results [21] a statistically significant difference was observed in terms of survival (p=0.039) in favour of primary chemotherapy, but with a longer follow-up (median 7 years) this difference disappeared. The breast conserving treatment rates after primary chemotherapy (82%) and after primary irradiation (77%) were equivalent and no difference in disease-free interval or local recurrence was observed.

St Petersburg trial [22]

The aim of this trial was to compare the efficacy of preoperative combined chemotherapy and irradiation with that of preoperative irradiation alone (Fig. 5). Pre- and postmenopausal women with clinical stage IIb-IIIa breast cancer were enrolled. Primary chemotherapy consisted of one or two courses of intramuscular thiotepa 20 mg on days 1, 3, 5, 7, 9 and 11, intravenous methotrexate 40 mg/m^2 on days 1 and 8, and intravenous 5FU 500 mg/m^2 on days 1 and 8. Locoregional treatment consisted of modified radical mastectomy in all cases, followed by four to six courses of adjuvant chemotherapy, which was identical to the primary chemotherapy. Histopathological assessment of the mastectomy

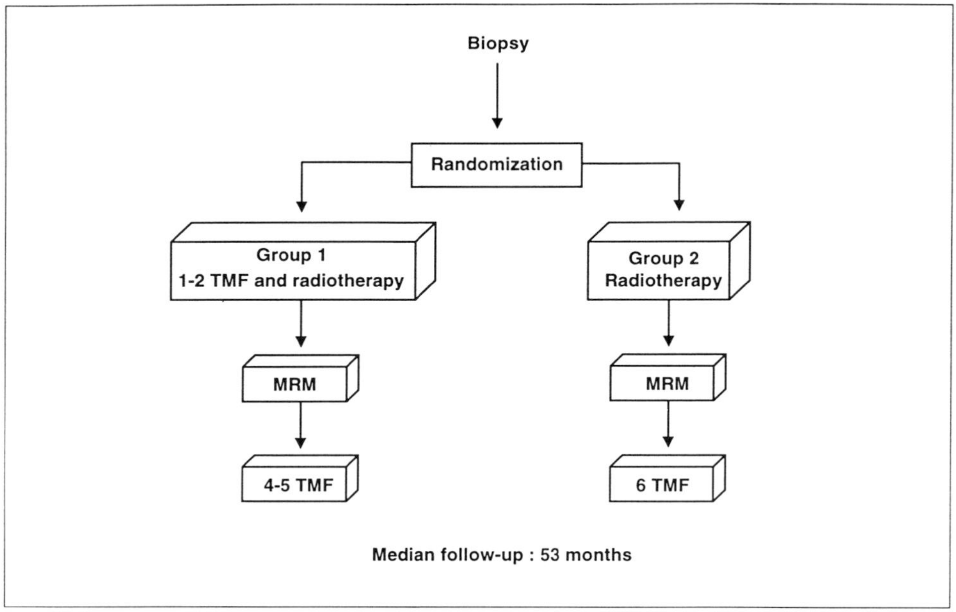

Fig. 5. Treatment schedule of St Petersburg trial.

specimens showed complete regression of the tumour in 29.1% after primary chemotherapy and in 19.4% after primary irradiation. The 5-year overall survival was identical in the two treatment groups, but the disease-free survival was better in the primary chemotherapy group (p=0.04).

Prediction of tumour response and outcome

Primary chemotherapy is an *in vivo* model where the informative value of a given tumour factor can be assessed simply by analysing tumour shrinkage. Pretherapeutic tumour core biopsy provides enough material to confirm the malignant and infiltrating nature of a breast tumour as well as to study and compare the predictive and prognostic values of different immunohistochemical factors. In the Institut Bergonié trial a retrospective analysis was performed on core biopsies of patients treated with primary chemotherapy [26]. We analysed 128 of the 134 tumour samples for 12 prognostic factors. Tumour size, SBR grade and DCC-ER were assessed in all cases. The other prognostic factors were analysed in 127 cases for DCC-PgR, in 126 cases for IHC-ER, Mib1 and GSTπ, in 125 cases for p53, c-erbB2 and pS2, in 124 cases for IHC-PgR. This difference was due to insufficient tumour material provided by initial biopsy.

Predictive factors for tumour response

Patients whose tumours were initially smaller than 4 cm were eligible for breast conserving treatment more frequently than those with larger tumours, but their regression rates during neoadjuvant chemotherapy were the same. ER/PgR+ tumours (tumours with one or two positive receptors) as detected by the biochemical assay had a lower rate of breast conserving treatment (52%) than ER/PgR− tumours (tumours with two negative receptors) (77%) because of the better regression of ER/PgR− tumours. The same result was shown retrospectively with IHC analysis of ER status but not of PgR status (curves not shown).

Ki67, a cell cycle nuclear protein associated with tumour proliferation, was assessed by IHC, using the Mib1 antibody [26]. Tumours which expressed Mib1 in more than 40% of cells showed better regression under neoadjuvant chemotherapy.

Multivariate analysis using logistic regression was done on 12 prognostic factors in order to predict the likelihood of obtaining a response rate greater than 50%: tumour size >40 mm, SBR grade 3, SBR grade 1, IHC-ER <10%, IHC-PgR <10%, DCC-ER <10 fmol/mg protein^{-1}, DCC-PgR <15 fmol/mg protein^{-1}, Mib1 >40%, pS2 <3%, p53 <0%, c-erbB2 <1 and glutathione-S-transferase pi (GSTπ) >1%. The three predictive factors in univariate analysis keep their independent informative values: tumours of smaller size, without any ER/PgR and with a high Mib1 expression have a better chance of being eligible for breast conserving treatment than the other tumours.

Prognostic factors for survival

Classical factors such as age, tumour size, response to neoadjuvant chemotherapy, SBR grade and ER/PgR status were not predictive of a good or poor survival irrespective of the treatment applied in groups A and B.

In the IHC retrospective study, univariate analysis showed that DCC and IHC-PgR negativity is predictive of poor overall survival (p=0.03; p=0.05) and Mib1 >40% is predictive of metastasis-free survival (p=0.05). Moreover, c-erbB2 positivity is predictive of poor disease-free, metastasis-free and overall survival (p=0.03; p=0.008; p=0.0006). In Cox's multivariate analysis including the 12 factors studied above, c-erbB2 >0% remains predictive of a poor overall survival (p=0.01) and of metastasis-free survival (p=0.01).

Conclusions

European trials have greatly contributed to the introduction of primary chemotherapy in current practice. After locally advanced and inflammatory breast cancers, operable breast tumours can be safely treated with primary chemotherapy. The optimal regimen to obtain the highest response rate has not yet been determined. The association of anthracyclines and taxanes is probably the most promising choice. Primary chemotherapy keeps its adjuvant efficacy but does not improve overall survival in comparison with classical adjuvant chemotherapy, despite the downstaging of nodal involvement as shown by the NSABP-B18 trial [27]. Several questions are still unanswered; they concern the association of endocrine and chemotherapy and the use of adjuvant chemotherapy after primary chemotherapy and locoregional treatment in case of persistence of bad prognostic factors (residual infiltrating tumour, high nodal involvement).

References

1   Haagensen CD, Stout AP. Carcinoma of the breast. II. Criteria of operability. Ann Surg 1943; 118: 859-70; 1032-51.
2   Fisher B, Saffer EA, Rudock C et al. Effect of local or systemic treatment prior to primary tumor removal on the production and response to a serum growth stimulating factor in mice. Cancer Res 1989; 49: 2002-4.
3   Fisher B, Saffer EA, Rudock C et al. Presence of a growth stimulating factor in serum following primary tumor removal in mice. Cancer Res 1989; 49: 1996-2001.
4   Goldie JH, Coldman AJ. A mathematical model for relating the drug sensitivity of tumors to their spontaneous mutation rate. Cancer Treat Rep 1979; 63: 1727-33.
5   Goldie JH, Coldman AJ. Quantitative model for multiple levels of drug resistance in clinical tumours. Cancer Treat Rep 1983; 67: 923-31.
6   Mauriac L. Chimiothérapie première des cancers du sein. Bull Cancer/Radiother 1995; 82: 158-67.
7   Chevallier B. Le cancer du sein inflammatoire. Bull Cancer 1993; 80: 1024-34.
8   Gisselbrecht C, Lepage E, Extra JM et al. Cancer du sein: traitement intensif avec autogreffe de moelle. Bull Cancer 1989; 76: 99-104.
9   Therasse P, Mauriac L, Welnicka M et al. Neo-adjuvant dose intensive chemotherapy in locally advanced breast cancer (LABC): an EORTC-NCIC-SAKK randomized phase III study comparing FEC (5FU, epirubicin, cyclophosphamide) vs high dose intensity EC + G-CSF (filgrastim). Am Soc Clin Oncol 1998; 17: 124 (abstract 472).
10   Lemaire M, Focan C, Desaive C et al. Neoadjuvant chemotherapy, with mitoxantrone, cyclophosphamide and fluorouracil in operable breast cancer of intermediate stage: first results of a phase II study in 40 patients. Bull Cancer 1992; 79: 883-91.
11   Belembaogo E, Feillel V, Chollet P et al. Neoadjuvant chemotherapy in 126 operable breast cancers. Eur J Cancer 1992; 28A: 896-900.
12   Calais G, Berger C, Descamps P et al. Conservative treatment feasibility with induction chemotherapy, surgery and radiotherapy for patients with breast carcinoma larger than 3 cm. Cancer 1994; 74: 1283-8.
13   Dieras V, Fumoleau P, Romieu G et al. A randomized, parallel study of doxorubicin/Taxol® (paclitaxel) and doxorubicin/cyclophosphamide as adjuvant treatment of breast cancer. Breast Cancer Res Treat 1998; 50 (abstract 25).
14   Chollet P, Charrier S, Brain E et al. Clinical and pathological response to primary chemotherapy in operable breast cancer. Eur J Cancer 1997; 33: 862-6.
15   Jacquillat C, Baillet F, Auclerc G et al. Cancer du sein. Chimiothérapie précédant le traitement loco-régional avec extension des indications du traitement conservateur. Sem Hôp Paris 1985; 61: 1452-6.
16   Bonadonna G, Valagussa P, Brambilla C et al. Primary chemotherapy in operable breast cancer: eight-year experience at the Milan Cancer Institute. J Clin Oncol 1998; 16: 93-100.

17 Cameron DA, Anderson EDC, Levack P et al. Primary systemic therapy for operable breast cancer. 10-year survival data after chemotherapy and hormone therapy. Br J Cancer 1997; 76: 1099-105.
18 Smith IE, Walsh G, Jones A et al. High complete remission rates with primary neoadjuvant infusional chemotherapy for large early breast cancer. J Clin Oncol 1995; 13: 424-9.
19 Mauriac L, Durand M, Avril A et al. Effects of primary chemotherapy in conservative treatment of breast cancer patients with operable tumors larger than 3 cm. Ann Oncol 1991; 2: 347-54.
20 Mauriac L, MacGrogan G, Avril A et al. Neoadjuvant chemotheapy for operable breast carcinoma larger than 3 cm: a unicentre randomized trial with a 124-month median follow-up. Ann Oncol 1999; 10: 47-52.
21 Scholl SM, Fourquet A, Asselain B et al. Neoadjuvant versus adjuvant chemotherapy in premenopausal patients with tumors considered too large for breast conserving surgery: preliminary results of a randomised trial: S6. Eur J Cancer 1994; 30A: 645-52.
22 Semiglazov VF, Topuzov EE, Bavli JL et al. Primary (neoadjuvant) chemotherapy and radiotherapy compared with primary radiotherapy alone in stage IIb-IIIa breast cancer. Ann Oncol 1994; 5: 591-5.
23 Makris A, Powles TJ, Ashley SE et al. A reduction in the requirements for mastectomy in a randomized trial of neoadjuvant chemoendocrine therapy in primary breast cancer. Ann Oncol 1998; 9: 1179-84.
24 Mauriac L, Wafflart J, Durand M et al. Apport de la drill-biopsie dans le bilan pré-thérapeutique des adénocarcinomes mammaires. Bull Cancer (Paris) 1981; 68: 417-21.
25 Mamounas EP. Preoperative chemotherapy: a model for studying the biology and therapy of primary breast cancer. J Clin Oncol 1995; 13: 537-40.
26 MacGrogan G, Mauriac L, Durand M et al. Primary chemotherapy in breast invasive carcinoma: predictive value of the immuno-histochemical detection of hormonal receptors, p53, c-erb-B2, MiB1, pS2 and GSTπ. Br J Cancer 1996; 74: 1458-65.
27 Fisher B, Brown A, Mamounas E et al. Effect of preoperative chemotherapy on local-regional disease in women with operable breast cancer: findings from National Surgical Adjuvant Breast and Bowel Project B-18. J Clin Oncol 1997; 15: 2483-93.

ESO Scientific Updates, Vol. 4
Primary Medical Therapy for Breast Cancer
A. Howell and M. Dowsett, editors
© 1999 Elsevier Science B.V. All rights reserved

The Primary Use of Endocrine Therapies

Anthony Howell[1] and John F.R. Robertson[2]

1   CRC Department of Medical Oncology, Christie Hospital NHS Trust, University of
    Manchester, United Kingdom
2   Department of Surgery, City Hospital, University of Nottingham, United Kingdom

Introduction

Endocrine therapy for advanced breast cancer and in the adjuvant situation is
well established; however, the first primary endocrine therapy trial using tamoxifen was not published until 1982 [1]. Since then a further eleven phase II
and III randomised trials have been published. In nearly all the phase II studies primary treatment was given to avoid an operation in elderly women who
were too infirm for surgery or refused it. We review the problems of this approach in the elderly and discuss how we might define the place of primary endocrine therapy in breast conservation and whether such treatment affects survival compared with postoperative treatment. Compared with primary chemotherapy, primary endocrine therapy can be given throughout the surgical period and the clinical potential of this approach needs to be explored together
with studies which define the value of the new antioestrogens and aromatase
inhibitors in this clinical situation. Here we will review the phase II and
phase III studies already published and indicate what we can learn from them
to design more definitive studies of primary endocrine therapy.

Phase II studies

Twelve phase II studies using endocrine therapy as primary treatment have
been reported. The rationale of systemic rather than surgical treatment was
that elderly women are frightened of hospitals, often have intercurrent illness
which makes surgery hazardous, and may die of another cause if tamoxifen controlled their tumour in the long term. In the first study Preece et al. [1] treated

---

Address for correspondence: A. Howell, CRC Department of Medical Oncology, Christie
Hospital NHS Trust, University of Manchester, Wilmslow Road, Manchester M20 4BX,
United Kingdom. Tel.: +44-161-4463746, fax: +44-161-4463299

67 women with stage II and III tumours over the age of 75 years. Forty-nine patients (73%) responded sufficiently to persist with treatment beyond the first follow-up visit. The authors pointed out that more than 12 months were required for 18% of tumours to achieve their ultimate response.

In the second reported study from Sweden the authors treated 26 women over the age of 65 years with 27 (1 bilateral) stage I and II tumours who were too infirm for surgery or who refused operation [2]. All tumours were 20 mm or less in diameter measured radiographically and the tumour volume change was computed from changes in mammographic size. Volume changes were used as the authors pointed out a reduction in diameter from 20 mm to 10 mm represents a volume change from 4200 mm^3 to 500 mm^3, which is nearly a 90% reduction. (By UICC criteria, where two diameters are multiplied, this would represent a 75% reduction). There was complete radiological remission in 15 tumours (56%) and six (22%) had 50% or more volume reduction. The follow-up time after complete remission was one to 26 months – none of the responding tumours regrew during this time. This study is important in showing a high CR rate (15 of 27) in small mammographically detected tumours unselected by ER measurement. In responders the time to achieve half volume ranged between 0.5 and 11.4 months, with a median of 1.5 months.

A larger study [3] treated 161 patients over the age of 70 with T1-T3 tumours. Evaluation was by means of calliper measurements and UICC criteria for response were used. Forty-four patients (27%) had a CR, 55 (34%) a PR, 39 (24%) were stable and 23 (14%) progressed immediately. There was no relationship between tumour size and response. Of the 99 patients who responded to treatment, 78% had done so by six months but a few took up to two years to attain their final response. Interpretation of the duration of response is complicated because during the first two years of the study tamoxifen was stopped after complete regression was obtained.

A study of 53 patients over the age of 60 with T1-T3 tumours [4] reported 29 (55%) of patients with a CR, 14 (26%) with a PR and 6 (11%) with stable disease; the overall response rate was thus 92%. This was the first study where oestrogen receptors were measured in a subset of patients. Two of 37 patients had ER-poor tumours and neither responded. The authors emphasised the slow time to response on tamoxifen with a median of 15.5 weeks.

Thirty patients over the age of 78 who were given primary tamoxifen treatment were reported by Margolese and Foster [5]. The results were reported as "50% reduction of the longest diameter" of the tumour. Five (17%) had a CR, 14 a PR (46%) and eight (27%) stabilisation for an overall response rate of 91%.

A very careful study of endocrine therapy in 61 patients with tumours >4 cm (age range 33-69 years) was reported by the Edinburgh group [6,7]. The first 36 patients were given various forms of endocrine therapy (5 oophorectomy, 17 goserelin, 10 aminoglutethimide and 11 tamoxifen). Following the demonstration that there were no responses in tumours with ER <20 fmol mg/cytosol protein a further 25 patients with ER+ tumours were treated with goserelin (n=9) or aminoglutethimide (n=16), depending on their menopausal status. Patients were reviewed weekly by a single member of the team and measurements were made in eight diameters with callipers. Mammograms were performed every month. Twenty-four of the 61 patients (39%) had significant tumour regression. There were no differences in the chances of regression with respect to menopausal status or type of endocrine therapy. In responders the median time to achieve half volume was 44 days (range 3-150 days). Since surgery was performed after three months of primary therapy it is not known whether longer treatment would have led to a higher response rate.

In a study of 40 patients over 67 years of age with 42 T1-T3 tumours Foudraine et al. [8] reported "remissions" in 17 (42.5%) and stable disease in 16 (40%) [8]. The mean time to remission was 8.9 months. Follow-up was relatively short at a mean of 25 months.

A further study was reported from Edinburgh [9] in a group of 66 patients ≥70 years of age. This study is also important because of the careful measurement of response. Calliper measurements of the tumour were performed four times during the first 12 weeks of treatment. A significant response was defined as a probability of greater than 95% that the regression line for tumour volume deviated from the horizontal. However, at three months this occurred in only 19 (29%) of patients. By UICC criteria 14 patients (21%) had a CR, 20 (30%) a PR and 5 (8%) stable disease. This group also defined "worthwhile response at two years", meaning that patients remained in remission at that time. The sensitivity and specificity of the prediction of "worthwhile" response is shown in Table 1 according to the method of prediction used, UICC criteria at six months, sequential measurements at three months and ER estimations. ER (≥20% of cells positive) had the greatest sensitivity but no method was particularly specific. This study also estimated the number of patients whose disease was controlled to death, which was 54%.

Table 1. Prediction of outcome of treatment at 2 years ("worthwhile response") by three different methods: sensitivity and specificity (from ref. 9)

Method	No. of pts	Predicted "worthwhile response"	Sensitivity (%)	Predicted failure	Specificity (%)
UICC six months	59	16 of 32	50	18 of 27	67
Sequential measurements for 3 months	59	21 of 32	66	12 of 27	44
Oestrogen receptor (≥ 20% cells stained)	47	26 of 27	96	12 of 20	60

A Dutch group [10] reported results in 34 patients aged 70 years or more with stage I-II breast cancer given tamoxifen alone. Twenty-five had what was described as good local control. The mean time to progression in nine patients was 21 months (range 2-151 months).

The Amsterdam/Rotterdam Group [11] assessed primary tamoxifen therapy in 85 patients 75 years or older. Disease was assessed by palpation and by mammography, according to UICC criteria. In 83 patients the reasons mentioned in the medical records for non-surgery were related to physical or mental condition (n=32), age alone (n=31), patient preference (n=30), and other reasons (n=20). Median follow-up was 28 months. Twelve patients had a CR (14%), 20 a PR (23%) and 39 were stable (46%). The median time to CR or PR was 6-7 months. Overall, 37 (43.5%) of patients showed tumour progression (always in the breast) during tamoxifen treatment, 24 of whom had a PR or stabilisation. Forty-five percent of patients were free of local progression at four years. Twenty of 37 (59%) patients were unfit for surgery at the time of progression; 14 of them had been fit at diagnosis. The authors could find no explanation of the relatively low response rate (37.6% CR and PR) compared with other studies.

A group from Florence [12] reported on the results of primary endocrine therapy with tamoxifen in 120 patients with T1-T4 tumours aged 70 and above: only 12 had T4 tumours and are included here, because it was not possible to assess the operable cancers separately. Tumour response was assessed by mammography according to UICC criteria at one, two and three months and then three-monthly. Complete remissions were seen in 12 (10%), PRs in 46 (38%) and stable disease in 53 (44%) patients.

In the majority of the studies above (with one exception [7] where goserelin and aminoglutethimide were used) tamoxifen was the endocrine therapy of choice. More recently, Dixon et al. [13] assessed the aromatase inhibitor letrozole (2.5 mg and 10 mg) in 24 patients aged between 61 and 87 years with tumours >3 cm and ER positive. Four patients had a CR, 18 a PR and two static disease, giving an overall response rate of 92%. Fifteen patients were estimated to require mastectomy but after therapy were able to have conservation surgery.

Randomised studies

Four randomised trials comparing preoperative tamoxifen with surgery have been previously reported. In two the comparison arm was surgery alone [14,15] and in the other two the comparison arm was surgery and adjuvant tamoxifen in addition [16,17]. All four studies were performed in elderly patients and mainly in those with T2 tumours (Table 2). Follow-up was shortest in the Italian GRETA trial. An overview of the CRC and GRETA trials was recently published in abstract form [18].

The local and distant relapse rates and survival of patients in the four trials are outlined in Table 3. The first Nottingham study [14] and the Gazet trial [15] had unexpectedly high local relapse rates in the surgery alone arms. This may

Table 2. Details of the four randomised trials where preoperative tamoxifen was compared with surgery with or without postoperative tamoxifen

Study	Treatment	Patients (n)	Age	Tumour eligibility	Median follow-up (months)	Median time to progression (months)
Robertson et al. [14]	Preop Tam Surgery	68 67	≥70	T1, T2	65	24 Not reached
Gazet et al. [15]	Preop Tam Surgery	100 100	≥70	T1-T4	72 (mean)	36 (approx.) 39 (approx.)
Bates et al. [16]	Preop Tam Surg + Tam	228 219	≥70	T1-T4	72	30 72
Mustacchi et al. [17]	Preop Tam Surg + Tam	236 237	≥65	T1-T3	37	45 Not reached

Table 3. Local and distant relapse rates and patient survival in the four randomised trials of preoperative endocrine therapy

Treatments tested	Local relapse		Distant relapse		Study
	T (%)	S±T (%)	T (%)	S±T (%)	
TvS	40/68 (59)	20/67 (30)	16/68 (24)	22/67 (34)	Robertson et al. [14]
TvS	56/100 (56)	44/100 (44)	8/100 (8)	14/100 (14)	Gazet et al. [15]
TvS+T	51/183 (28)	22/177 (12)	6/183 (3)	6/171 (3)	Bates el al. [16]
TvS+T	60/236 (25)	15/237 (6)	19/236 (8)	33/237 (14)	Mustacchi et al. [17]
	Deaths from breast cancer		*Deaths from other causes*		
TvS	15/168 (22)	16/67 (24)	13/68 (19)	12/67 (18)	Robertson et al. [14]
TvS	17/100 (17)	13/100 (13)	16/100 (16)	13/100 (13)	Gazet et al. [15]
TvS+T	18/236 (7)	27/237 (11)	23/236 (10)	21/237 (9)	Mustacchi et al. [17]

T, tamoxifen; S, surgery

be explained by the fact that in the Nottingham study surgery consisted of a wedge mastectomy while in the Gazet study some patients with stage III tumours received breast conservation. Also in the Nottingham study axillary lymph nodes were only resected if symptomatic. Despite this, local relapse (in the breast) in the tamoxifen arm was even higher than in the surgery arm. Comparison of local recurrence rates by treatment in the first Nottingham study is shown in Figure 1. Local relapse rates in the CRC and GRETA trials in the surgery arm were lower, possibly because of the use of postoperative tamoxifen. At the time of analysis about one quarter of patients had relapsed locally in the primary tamoxifen-treated groups. Paradoxically, there were fewer distant relapses in the primary tamoxifen groups in three of the four trials (Table 3). There were no significant differences in deaths from breast cancer or from other causes in the three trials where this was reported. In the recent overview of the CRC and GRETA trials there was a survival advantage for women treated by surgery but this was not significant at the conventional level (RR 0.86; p=0.09) [18]. However, there was a significant difference in favour of the surgically treated group in terms of breast cancer deaths.

There is one further randomised study (from Nottingham) of tamoxifen versus surgery plus adjuvant tamoxifen as primary treatment in elderly patients. The randomised comparison has yet to be reported. However, in the tamoxifen-treated arm the response results by the ER measurements in the primary tumour have been reported [19]. This latter publication showed high initial response rates in those tumours (median for 13 months) where the ER H-score was greater than 100. The conclusion was made that H-score could be used to select patients for preoperative tamoxifen treatment. The difference between the two Nottingham studies in terms of the tamoxifen arm was that in the first study there was no selection on the basis of ER whereas there was in the second (H-score >100). If one removes the patients who progressed *de novo* (within six months) in the first study and then plots the time-to-progression curves from the two studies, the results overlap (Fig. 2). Therefore, while ER may help exclude patients, some of whom may have benefitted from an endocrine agent, the duration of response is the same as for patients without ER status.

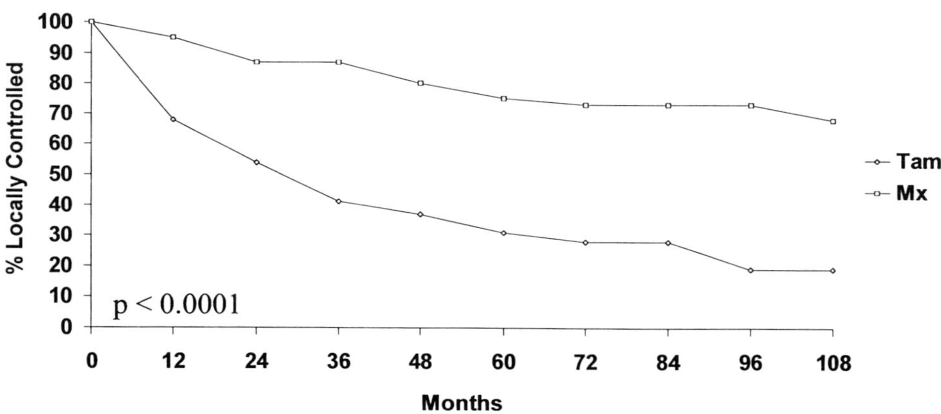

Fig. 1. Comparison of local recurrence rates by primary treatment in the first Nottingham study.

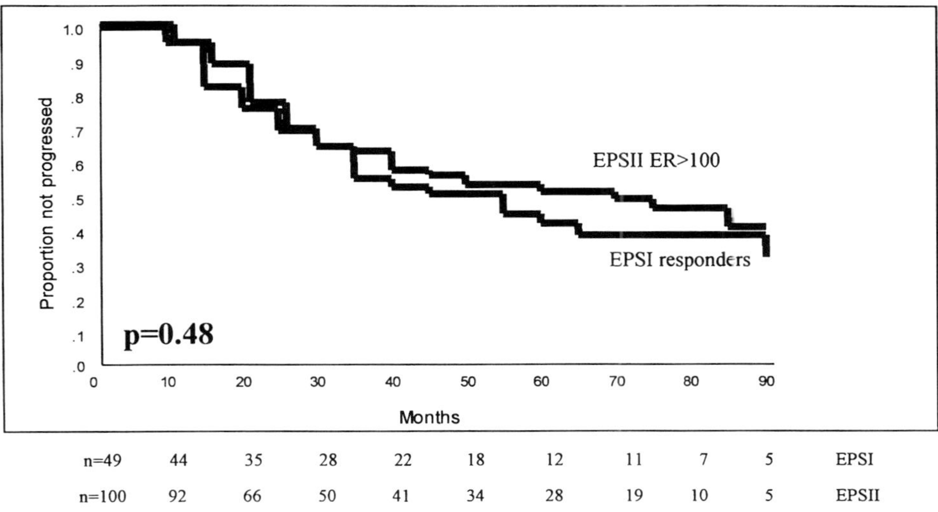

Fig. 2. Time to progression curves from the first (EPSI) and second (EPSII) Nottingham studies. Local control on primary tamoxifen; EPSI responders vs EPSII ER>100.

Comments on the phase II and randomised trials

The percentage of breast cancers which express oestrogen receptors increases with the age of the patient [14,20]. The phase II studies included mainly elderly, unfit patients. It is not surprising therefore that high response rates were reported in these studies. What is more interesting is that, despite the high ER and despite the unfit elderly population, tamoxifen did not control the majority of cancers.

The average life expectancy of women at 70 is 15 years. Allowing for the fact that the phase II studies were mainly in a sub-population of older, medically unfit patients, it is not surprising that, when tamoxifen was compared with surgery in randomised studies, there was a significantly higher local failure rate in the tamoxifen arm of the Nottingham study, as shown in Figure 1. There was no difference in local recurrence in the Gazet study, but this is most likely to be due to the fact that some patients may have received inadequate surgery (e.g. wide local excision for stage III cancers).

There have been three randomised studies of tamoxifen versus surgery plus tamoxifen. Two have reported the initial results (CRC and GRETA trials), again showing a significantly higher local failure rate in the tamoxifen arms. Neither of these studies selected patients on the basis of ER. A third randomised study of tamoxifen versus tamoxifen plus surgery which did select patients on the basis of high ER (H-score >100) has yet to report results of the randomised comparison. Initial results showing very high response rates and better duration of response have been reported [19].

The recent combined analysis of the CRC and GRETA [18] trials reported that the difference in survival almost reached statistical significance (p=0.09) in favour of the surgery plus tamoxifen arm and that the difference in breast cancer deaths was statistically significant. The second Nottingham trial also is starting to show a divergence of the survival curves at four years in favour of the surgery plus tamoxifen arm (personal communication). These data would suggest that elderly patients should receive standard therapy (i.e. surgery plus adjuvant therapy) until studies of sufficient power show that tamoxifen alone is equivalent. Furthermore, in using tamoxifen as first-line therapy a number of elderly patients fit for surgery become unfit for surgery by the time they progress on tamoxifen. Another point to be considered is that because of the high local failure rate on tamoxifen it would be essential that such patients be seen regularly for clinical examination (probably three-monthly at least for the first two years and six-monthly thereafter). This is exactly the population of patients (i.e. elderly unfit) who are least able to make regular, repeated outpatient visits.

Response rates to primary endocrine therapy

Figure 3 summarises the reported response rates in 12 phase II trials and the primary tamoxifen arms of the four randomised trials. Complete response rates varied from 8% to 58%, partial response rates from 15% to 75%, stable disease from 7% to 50%, and progressive disease from 0% to 23%. In most studies treatment was not selected on the basis of tumour ER or too few patients were selected in this way to affect, appreciably, the overall response assessment [7,11]. In a fifth randomised study which has yet to be reported all patients were selected on the basis of ER (H-score >100.) Of the first 50 patients who were treated with tamoxifen, 52% had a CR and 34% a PR [19].

The methods of evaluation of response included change in a single tumour diameter [8], change in the product of two diameters according to UICC criteria [3], halving of the volume [2], the slope of the regression curve of four measurements over a 12-week period [9] by mammography [12] and ultrasound [13]. All of these methods are likely to give different results from each other because of different changes in tumour volume required for inclusion in each response category. In addition, mammography is likely to produce fewer CRs even if the tumour is impalpable clinically since a small residium may be seen which could be classed as a PR. These studies and the variation shown highlight the need to have consistent response criteria for primary treatments in order to compare response rates between studies and between different endocrine agents.

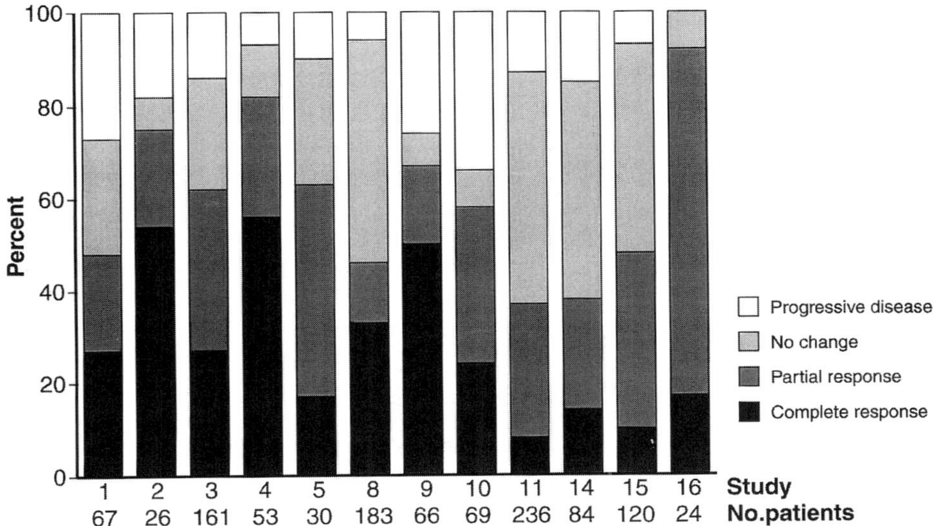

Fig. 3. Response categories after use of primary endocrine therapy in trials where these data were reported.

Time to response

The median time to CR in the relatively small number of studies where this was reported ranged from 5 to 27 months and for time to PR the range of medians was 3 to 10 months (Table 4). Not surprisingly, time to PR was shorter than time to CR. The time to CR was up to 34 months in one study and indicates the slowness with which some tumours respond. Also it is likely that length of time to mammographic CR will be longer than clinical CR [12]. The variation in time to response is also, in part, responsible for the variation in response rates between studies since it is clear that the proportions of subjects reported in each response category will depend upon the time from the start of tamoxifen when responses were evaluated. It will also depend on the assiduousness of follow-up. Since some of the studies outlined above were retrospective reviews the response rates are likely to be rough estimates.

Duration of response

In most studies primary endocrine therapy was given until tumour progression and so the duration of response could be assessed. The four studies where duration of response was assessed are outlined in Table 5. The median durations of CR ranged from 23 to 41 months, for PR the range was 12-30 months and for sta-

Table 4. Variation in time to maximum response in studies where this was assessed: figures are medians and, in brackets, ranges in months

Complete response	Partial response	Authors
14 (3-25)	-	Helleberg et al. 1982 [2]
5 (2-24)	3 (2-7)	Bradbeer & Kyngdon 1983 [3]
4 (1.5-34) (includes PR)		Allan et al. 1985 [4]
9 (?) (includes PR)		Foudraine et al. 1992 [8]
6 (1-24)	7 (2-26)	Bergman et al. 1995 [11]
27 (?)	10 (?)	Ciatto et al. 1996 [12]

Table 5. Duration of remission (months + range) according to response categories in studies where this was reported

Complete response	Partial response	Stable disease	Authors
24 (6-36+)	12 (6-36+)	12 (6-36+)	Preece et al. 1982 [1]
25 (2-60)	14 (2-60)	-	Bradbeer & Kyngdon 1983 [2]
23 (5-48)	14 (6-55)	15 (?)	Allan et al. 1985 [4]
41 (?)	30 (?)		Ciatto et al. 1996 [12]

ble disease 12-15 months. These figures are similar to those of studies of first-line endocrine therapy in advanced breast cancer. The majority of patients in the studies of primary endocrine therapy progressed within three years of initiation of endocrine therapy. This is similar to advanced breast cancer where the corresponding figure is two years. The difference in the median TTP values of studies of elderly patients with operable breast cancer and those with advanced breast cancer may be due to the higher expression of ER in tumours of elderly patients.

Prediction of response

Assessment of response at three or six months is, unfortunately, a poor predictor of the outcome at two years, as demonstrated in the Edinburgh study (Table 1). In this study, ER measurement had a sensitivity of 90% and a specificity of 60%, which is superior to methods using tumour measurement. It is likely that other methods such as short-term changes in tumour biochemistry [see chapters in this volume by Miller and Dowsett] may ultimately give improved prediction; however, at present oestrogen receptor gives the best indication, as shown in four studies summarised in Table 6.

Table 6. Response to primary endocrine therapy in patients with ER$^+$ tumours

Definition of receptor positivity	Patients (n)	CR + PR (%)	CR + PR + SD (%)	Authors
Score > 100	47	85	98	Low et al. 1992 [19]
>25% of cells positive	31	84	100	Gaskell et al. 1989 [28]
≥20% cells positive	34	79	91	Gaskell et al. 1992 [9]
Score > 80	24	92	100	Dixon et al. 1997 [13]

CR, complete response; PR, partial response; SD, stable disease

Problems with primary endocrine therapy in the elderly

Nearly all the phase II studies outlined above were pilot studies to determine the outcome of treating with primary endocrine therapy elderly patients who were either deemed to be unfit for surgery or refused operation. If a consensus can be reached it is that tamoxifen (which was used in all but two studies) may cause tumour regressions and thus delay the need for surgery. Many investigators point out that the survival of 70 or 80 year olds may be long and that in the majority of patients tumour control is lost before death, thus necessitating surgery at an older age. The randomised trials show that there is no definite survival disadvantage to the approach, although none of the studies were powered to show equivalence. However, the combined CRC/GRETA analysis shows a trend to reduced survival in the primary endocrine therapy treated patients [18] and a significantly lower number of deaths from breast cancer.

The phase II and randomised trials emphasise the difficulties of long-term primary endocrine therapy in the elderly. In contradistinction to primary surgery, women on tamoxifen have to be followed carefully to monitor progression and thus multiple visits to the hospital are required. There may also be problems of compliance with medication and loss to follow-up. Surgery is often required for local control later when patients are older and potentially more infirm. The general surgical consensus in the UK is for primary surgery to be performed wherever possible followed by adjuvant endocrine therapy, i.e., that elderly patients should not be treated differently from younger patients.

Rationale of primary endocrine therapy

The rationale of primary endocrine therapy has, to date, mainly been to avoid surgery in elderly patients. This rationale is different from the rationale for primary chemotherapy [see chapters by Assersohn and Powles and Mauriac et al. in this volume]. Initially, chemotherapy was used to downstage tumours in order to increase the chances of breast conservation. During these studies it was found that response was related to outcome and thus was a prognostic factor. Four randomised trials were performed in order to determine whether preoperative chemotherapy improved survival: they conclusively show that, with the chemotherapy currently available, there is no survival advantage to preoperative treatments.

Are any of the questions asked of primary chemotherapy (i.e., downstaging, prognosis, survival) answerable from the available data on primary endocrine therapy? The answer is a highly qualified "yes". One study has demonstrated that three months of primary letrozole allows downstaging of large ER-positive tumours in elderly women so that breast conservation may occur [13]. A further study [26] has recently reported that tamoxifen and gamma linoleic acid (GLA) in combination results in a rapid shrinkage of tumours: this is associated with a greater downregulation of ER expression than seen with tamoxifen alone. Two studies show that response to primary endocrine therapy is associated with improved survival compared with lack of response [3,11]. However, no studies have addressed the question of whether a fixed period (as used in primary chemotherapy studies) of primary endocrine therapy affects survival.

Future studies

The two major questions concerning primary endocrine therapy which have not been formally answered are:
1. Can tumours be safely downstaged by therapy?
2. Is there a survival advantage when endocrine therapy is used for a period preoperatively as well as postoperatively compared with postoperative use alone?

Downstaging

We might predict from all the response data outlined above that primary endocrine therapy will downstage the majority of ER-positive tumours. However, formal investigation of this approach in terms of allowing conservation therapy to be used safely has not been undertaken. It is likely that response followed by conservation surgery and postoperative radiation therapy will be safe, as has been shown for primary chemotherapy. However, it is possible that local control may be worse after primary endocrine therapy and formal studies to confirm or refute this conjecture are required. The questions then arise which endocrine therapy should be given and for how long.

It is clear that tamoxifen results in slower tumour regression than primary chemotherapy. Treatment may be required beyond six months and might be given up to the time of maximum regression as judged by serial calliper measurements, mammography or ultrasound. Furthermore, when does the clinician judge that the best response has been achieved and not wait too long until the tumour progresses? A highly important question is whether the new antioestrogens, such as Faslodex, or the new aromatase inhibitors, such as letrozole and anastrazole, induce more rapid responses, making downstaging with primary endocrine therapy more attractive.

Survival and primary endocrine therapy

Fisher and Mamounas [21] outlined possible reasons why primary therapy may improve survival. These include i) prevention of seeding of tumour cells shed at surgery, ii) inhibition of the release of growth stimulators of metastases from the primary tumour at surgery [22,23] and iii) prevention of drug resistance by immediate use of therapy [24]. In addition, it is known from animal experiments that inhibitors of angiogenesis are secreted by tumours [25]. If these are removed at surgery, remaining micrometastases may begin to grow. Most of the above arguments relate to the period of surgery. One advantage of primary endocrine therapy compared with primary chemotherapy is that the former may be continued throughout the surgical period. It is possible that a short period of endocrine therapy pre- and perioperatively will improve survival. Clearly this would not allow tumour downstaging. However, since the majority of tumours which present now are amenable to conservation surgery, this short treatment approach is attractive. Thus, two of several possible approaches to properly establishing the value of primary endocrine therapy might be:

- for large operable tumours: surgery → endocrine therapy versus endocrine therapy to maximum response → surgery → endocrine therapy;
- for tumours where conservation is feasible: surgery → endocrine therapy versus 2-4 weeks of pre and peri-operative endocrine therapy → surgery → endocrine therapy.

Summary

There remain a large number of outstanding questions concerning the value of primary endocrine therapy. Until now it may be argued that it is only appropriate treatment for women who are unfit for surgery and have ER-positive tumours.

Some of the outstanding questions concerning preoperative endocrine therapy include:

1. Can tumours be downstaged such that conservation therapy is safe?
2. Does appropriate primary endocrine therapy improve patient survival?
3. Should primary therapy be given for long or short periods?
4. Should the length of treatment depend upon the question being answered (e.g. conservation versus survival)?

5. Which are the most appropriate endocrine therapies to compare with tamoxifen as the gold standard (aromatase inhibitors, anastrozole and letrozole; new antioestrogens such as Faslodex and EM800 [27])?
6. Can we improve on ER to predict the most appropriate patients to treat?

Answers to these questions will come from innovative studies. Some of the background to this area is outlined in subsequent chapters.

References

1   Preece PE, Wood RA, Mackie CR et al. Tamoxifen as initial sole treatment of localised breast cancer in elderly women: a pilot study. Br Med J 1982; 284: 869-70
2   Helleberg A, Lundgren B, Norin T et al. Treatment of early localized breast cancer in elderly patients by tamoxifen. Br J Radiol 1982; 55: 511-5
3   Bradbeer JW, Kyngdon J. Primary treatment of breast cancer in elderly women with tamoxifen. Clin Oncol 1983; 9: 31-4
4   Allan SG, Rodger A, Smyth JF et al. Tamoxifen as primary treatment of breast cancer in elderly or frail patients: a practical management. Br Med J 1985; 290: 358
5   Margolese RG, Foster RS. Tamoxifen as an alternative to surgical resection for selected geriatric patients with primary breast cancer. Arch Surg 1989; 124: 548-50
6   Anderson EDC, Forrest APM, Levack PA et al. Response to endocrine manipulation and oestrogen receptor concentration in large operable breast cancer. Br J Cancer 1989; 60: 223
7   Anderson EDC, Forrest AP, Hawkins RA et al. Primary systemic therapy for operable breast cancer. Br J Cancer 1991; 63: 561-6
8   Foudraine NA, Verhoef LCG, Burghouts JT. Tamoxifen as sole therapy for primary breast cancer in the elderly patient. Eur J Cancer 1992; 28A; 900-3
9   Gaskell DJ, Hawkins RA, deCarteret S et al. Indications for primary tamoxifen therapy in elderly women with breast cancer. Br J Surg 1992; 79: 1317-20
10   van Dalsen AD, deVries JE. Treatment of breast cancer in elderly patients. J Surg Oncol 1995; 60: 80-2
11   Bergman L, van Dongen JA, van Ooijen B et al. Should tamoxifen be a primary treatment choice for elderly breast cancer patients with locoregional disease? Breast Cancer Res Treat 1995; 34: 77-83
12   Ciatto S, Cirillo A, Confortini M, DeLuca Cardillo C. Tamoxifen as primary treatment of breast cancer in elderly patients. Neoplasma 1996; 43: 43-5
13   Dixon JM, Love CDB, Tucker S et al. Letrozole as primary medical therapy for locally advanced and large operable breast cancer. Breast Cancer Res Treat 1997; 46: 213
14   Robertson JFR, Ellis IO, Elston CW et al. Mastectomy or tamoxifen as initial therapy for operable breast cancer in elderly patients: 5 year follow-up. Eur J Cancer 1992; 28A: 908-10
15   Gazet JC, Ford HT, Coombes RC et al. Prospective randomized trial of tamoxifen vs surgery in elderly patients with breast cancer. Eur J Surg Oncol 1994; 20: 207-14
16   Bates T, Riley DL, Houghton J et al. Breast cancer in elderly women: a Cancer Research Campaign trial comparing treatment with tamoxifen and optimal surgery with tamoxifen alone. Br J Surg 1991; 78: 591-4
17   Mustacchi G, Milani S, Pluchinotta A et al. Tamoxifen or surgery plus tamoxifen as primary treatment for elderly patients with operable breast cancer: the GRETA trial. Anticancer Res 1994; 14: 2197-200

18 Mustacchi G, Latteier J, Baum M, Ceccherini R et al. Tamoxifen alone versus surgery plus tamoxifen for breast cancer of the elderly. Meta-analysis of long term results of the GRETA and CRC trials. Breast Cancer Res Treat 1998; 50: 227

19 Low SC, Dixon AR, Bell J et al. Tumor oestrogen receptor content allows selection of elderly patients with breast cancer for conservative tamoxifen treatment. Br J Surg 1992; 79: 1314-6

20 Thorpe SM. Estrogen and progesterone receptor determination in breast cancer. Acta Oncologica 1988; 27: 1-19

21 Fisher B, Mamounas EP. Preoperative chemotherapy: a model for studying the biology and therapy of primary breast cancer. J Clin Oncol 1995; 3: 537-40

22 Fisher B, Gunduz N, Coyle J et al. Presence of a growth-stimulating factor in serum following primary tumor removal in mice. Cancer Res 1989; 49: 1996-2001

23 Fisher B, Saffer E, Rudosch C et al. Effect of local or systemic treatment prior to primary tumor removal on the production and response to a serum growth-stimulating factor in mice. Cancer Res 1989; 49: 2002-4

24 Goldie JH, Coldman AJ. A mathematic model for relating the drug sensitivity of tumours to their spontaneous mutation rate. Cancer Treat Rep 1979; 63: 1727

25 Folkman J. The role of angiogenesis in tumour growth. Semin Cancer Biol 1992; 3: 65-71

26 Kenny FS, Pinder S, Ellis IO, Bryce RP, Robertson JFR. GLA with tamoxifen as primary therapy in breast cancer - early results of a phase II pilot study. Breast Cancer Res Treat 1998; 50: 306

27 Tremblay A, Tremblay GB, Labrie C, Labrie F, Giguere V. EM-800, a novel antiestrogen, acts as a pure antagonist of the transcriptonal functions of estrogen receptors alpha and beta. Endocrinology 1998; 139: 111-8

28 Gaskell DJ, Hawkins RA, Sangster K, Chetty U, Forrest APM. Relation between immunocytochemical estimation of oestrogen receptor in elderly patients with primary breast cancer and response to tamoxifen. Lancet 1989; 1: 1044-6

ESO Scientific Updates, Vol. 4
Primary Medical Therapy for Breast Cancer
A. Howell and M. Dowsett, editors
© 1999 Elsevier Science B.V. All rights reserved

Pitfalls and Problems in Primary Medical Therapy: A Surgical Perspective

Nigel J. Bundred, Galal AbouElnagah and Maria Bramley

Department of Academic Surgical Oncology, University Hospital of South Manchester, Manchester, United Kingdom

Introduction

The initial aim of primary medical therapy in the form of neoadjuvant or pre-operative chemotherapy was to improve survival and reduce the need for mastectomy [1-5]. Recent results from randomised studies indicate it is unlikely that at present there will be a survival benefit, although there is clearly a reduction in the need for mastectomy [2,4,5,8]. The aim of this chapter is to direct surgeons to the role of primary medical therapy (either endocrine or chemotherapy) and its value in achieving an increased rate of breast conservation.

Studies of primary chemotherapy have shown a 70-90% response rate, which is associated with an increased breast conservation (BC) rate and decreased pathological node involvement [2,4,5]. The National Surgical Adjuvant Breast and Bowel Project (NSABP) clinical trial B-18 evaluated the role of pre-operative chemotherapy in 1300 patients and demonstrated that there was a reduced need for mastectomy and a reduced incidence of nodal involvement [2]. At least three of the randomised controlled trials in the medical literature attest to these findings [2,4,5].

The second concept, that primary chemotherapy would provide early elimination of metastatic microfoci of disease and increase survival, does not appear to have been convincingly proven by the same trials. Consequently, there is a need to select patients who will benefit from primary chemotherapy and those who should have conventional surgery followed by adjuvant chemotherapy. In addition, we need to understand how primary and adjuvant medical therapy can be integrated in high risk breast cancer patients to significantly increase survival compared to our current approach.

Address for correspondence: N.J. Bundred, Department of Academic Surgical Oncology, University Hospital of South Manchester, Nell Lane, Manchester M20 8LR, United Kingdom. Tel.: +44-161-2913842, fax: +44-161-2913846, e-mail: bundredn@fs1.with.man.ac.uk

Whilst current or future randomised controlled trials may demonstrate a survival advantage to using primary medical therapy, until they do so, primary chemotherapy or endocrine therapy should be restricted, outside the context of a clinical trial, to those large tumours (>4 cm in size) for which breast conserving surgery would be inappropriate at presentation.

Suitability/Selection of patients

Most patients with breast cancer will be referred to a surgeon for diagnosis and it is important that the surgeon be familiar with the concept of neoadjuvant therapy and the indications for its use. The usual indication for mastectomy is breast cancers of greater than 4 cm in size or palpable axillary lymph nodes greater than 1 cm in size, and both of these are an indication for primary endocrine/chemotherapy [1-8]. However, patients who have gross multifocal disease in the breast or who have widespread microcalcification throughout the breast (indicative of ductal carcinoma *in situ*) will need mastectomy whether or not they respond to preoperative therapy and should undergo mastectomy [1, 10]. Consequently, selection of patients for primary medical therapy requires a mammogram at diagnosis. This will exclude the multifocal tumours in the same breast or widespread microcalcification, which precludes primary medical therapy (Fig. 1). Some would argue that strongly oestrogen receptor-positive tumours which may be suitable for primary endocrine therapy in the context of a randomised controlled trial should not be given chemotherapy preoperatively [6,7]. Another relative contraindication for primary medical therapy is previous ipsilateral radiotherapy to the breast, which precludes breast conserving surgery [1].

Once eligibility for primary medical therapy is established, at least half of all women invited to have primary chemotherapy will decline and opt for mastectomy. Usually decliners are older, postmenopausal and more concerned with the toxicity of chemotherapy.

Diagnosis

Many patients are now diagnosed as having breast cancer on cytological assessment. This is, however, an inappropriate selection procedure for primary chemotherapy as it does not exclude the possibility of ductal carcinoma *in situ*, which will not respond to primary chemotherapy [1,8]. It is therefore imperative that the initial diagnosis of patients who are going to undergo primary medical therapy should be by a thick needle biopsy (core or trucut). Such a diagnostic strategy not only provides histopathological confirmation of invasive cancer but also allows the cancer to be graded and assessment of biological parameters such as hormone receptor status and c-erbB2 oncogene expression [6,7]. In particular thick needle tissue biopsy excludes ductal carcinoma *in situ* and

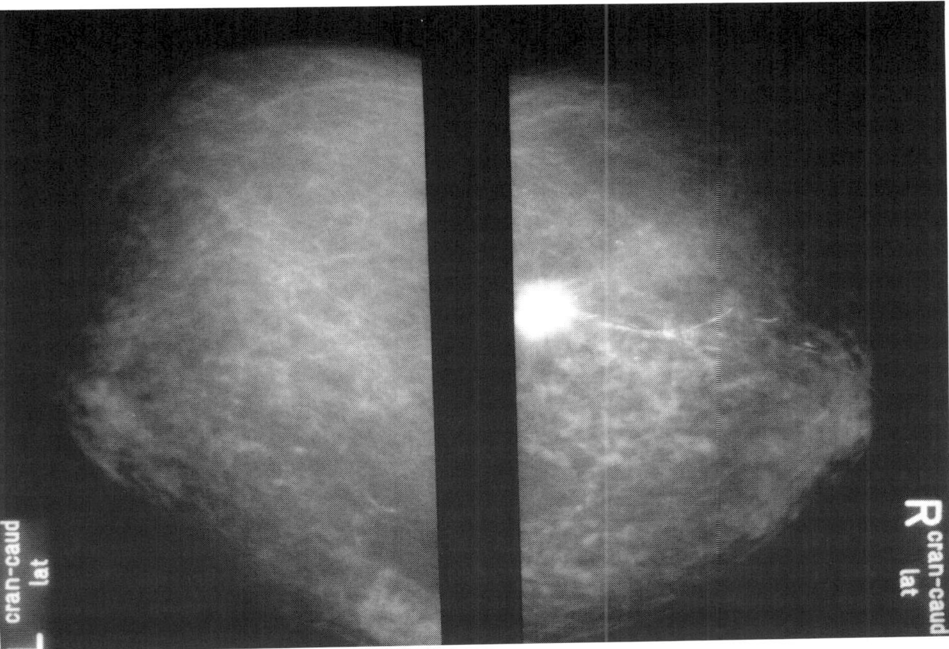

Fig. 1. Mammograms showing widespread microcalcification radiating out to the nipple from a tumour lying posterior in the breast on a cranio-caudal view right mammogram. Tumour needs mastectomy and the surrounding DCIS radiating to the nipple will not respond to primary medical therapy.

reduces the risk of overtreatment in the case of grade one, strongly oestrogen receptor-positive tumours. This is important since in one trial four out of 100 patients randomised underwent primary chemotherapy despite only having a diagnosis of ductal carcinoma *in situ* which (a) did not respond to the therapy (Fig. 2) , and (b) did not require the therapy [8]. In our experience and that of others [1,18] widespread ductal carcinoma *in situ* around a tumour requires mastectomy at presentation and it is therefore important to exclude this diagnosis. Another reason why initial thick needle biopsy is required for diagnosis is that potentially chemotherapy might change standard prognostic factors (e.g. ER status). After chemotherapy, node status is less often positive [2,4,5] and potentially it may also alter hormone receptor status and grade. Hawkins et al. found no change in oestrogen receptor concentration (as assessed by saturation analysis after primary chemotherapy) [11]. Thus there is a potential for standard prognostic factors to be altered by therapy and it is not clear whether the same significance can be attached to prognostic factors as is the case prior to chemotherapy. A thick needle biopsy allows measurement of a large number of these prognostic factors preoperatively (with the exception of node positivity)

Mammographic Reduction in
Tumour Volume with Chemotherapy

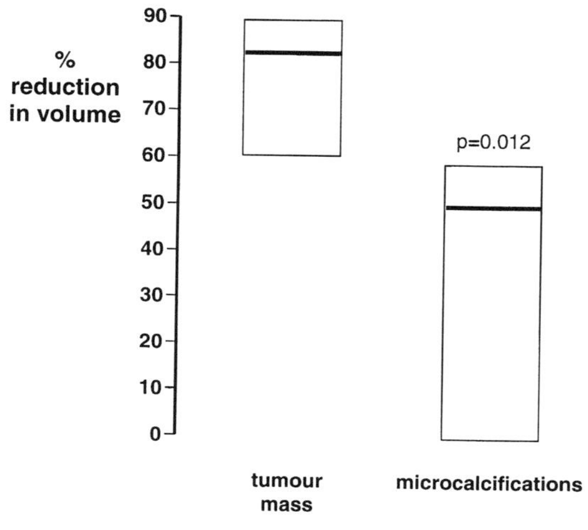

Fig. 2. Results from 107 women treated with primary chemotherapy in Manchester; 80% responded to chemotherapy with a reduction in tumour volume but less than 50% of those with microcalcification surrounding the tumour (rather than within the tumour) responded, indicating that ductal carcinoma *in situ* does not tend to respond to chemotherapy.

and helps to predict overall survival. We are aware that in a regional centre it is easy to fail to carry out either trucut biopsy or mammograms pre-therapy as patients will often have been diagnosed in another hospital, but we feel it is imperative that a thick needle biopsy, mammograms and an ultrasound [9] of the cancer are performed before chemotherapy is commenced.

Prediction of response

Non-responders account for 10-20% of women treated with primary medical therapy [1-6]. The ability to identify this group of women (in advance or early in treatment) would allow alternative treatment strategies. The Edinburgh group used endocrine therapy if the oestrogen receptor level was greater than 20 fmol/mg protein and reserved chemotherapy for those judged oestrogen receptor negative (less than 20 fmol/mg protein) [6]. They also gave chemotherapy to non-responders who were originally treated with endocrine therapy. A response was observed in 39% (24/61) patients who received primary endocrine therapy compared to a response rate of 72% following primary chemotherapy. In this study it is important to recognise that the median time taken to halve the tumour volume in the endocrine group was 44 days (range 3-150 days), which was almost twice as long as that for cytotoxic therapy at 20 days (range 3-77) (Fig. 3).

Mansi et al. found a 47% response rate to endocrine therapy and a 60% response rate to chemotherapy in 57 women with large tumours treated by primary medical therapy [12]. In addition, treatment with some endocrine agents (e.g. tamoxifen) does not reliably cause tumour regression but often produced long-term tumour stasis (stable disease). It is notable that response rates (CR and PR) to primary endocrine therapy in young women (<60 years of age) are less than the 61-73% reported response rates in women >70 years of age [13]. This may be because many studies of primary medical therapy in the elderly have continued endocrine treatment until evidence of relapse at a median of 3.5 years [13] rather than reporting clinical response after 6 months' treatment.

MacGrogan et al. used primary chemotherapy and found that the presence of a negative oestrogen receptor status, a high Mib1 (>40%) and a large tumour size predicted response to therapy [7]. It should be noted that a Mib1 of >40% is well above the median normally recorded in most laboratories [14].

It is generally accepted that, whether endocrine or chemotherapy is chosen for the first three months, no change of therapy should occur unless there are signs of progression (breast lymphoedema or increase in tumour size >25% according to UICC) which should lead to consideration for change of therapy [1, 6].

Interestingly, there are at least two studies which suggest that, although the presence of c-erbB2 oncogene does not predict for response to chemotherapy, it does predict for disease-free interval and overall survival [7]. This would appear to confirm the perception that expression of c-erbB2 oncogene allows early tumour regrowth and metastasis. More recently, American investigators have claimed c-erbB2 expression predicts response to adriamycin-containing chemotherapy regimens but not to other chemotherapeutic agents [15]. The hypothesis requires testing in a neoadjuvant setting. The presence of positive axillary nodes after medical therapy and surgery presents us with a challenging clinical scenario. Clinical trials are required to clarify what, if any, adjuvant therapy should be given to such node-positive women. Is this a setting which should be used to test novel therapeutic agents (i.e. antiangiogenic therapy)? If one undergoes neoadjuvant chemotherapy to achieve breast conservation (BC), the best marker of response allowing conservation is initial tumour size. Ninety-eight percent of tumours initially 3-4 cm in size shrink to allow BC compared to 27% of tumours originally 6-7 cm in size [1,2].

Assessment of response

Assessment of response has traditionally been clinicopathological and radiological [1,8]. Complete clinical response means there is no radiological or clini-

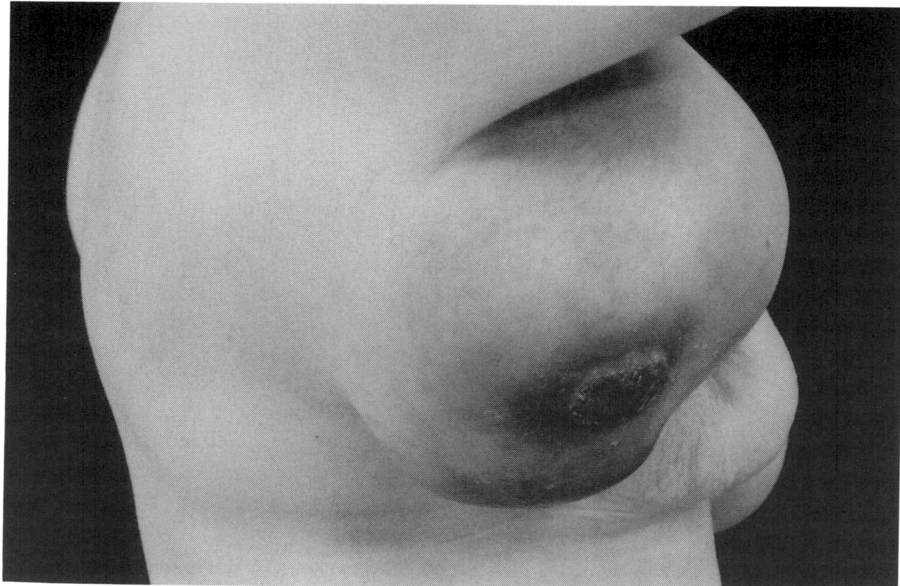

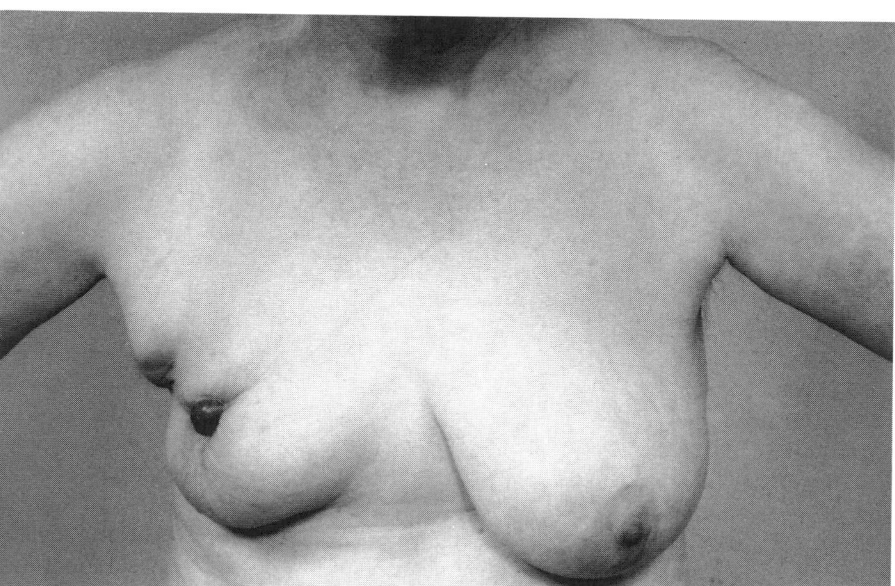

Fig. 3. (a) A 60-year-old lady presenting with a large mass in the axilla and a T4 carcinoma in the right breast. (b) Same lady at six months' treatment with tamoxifen demonstrating good response of the axillary tumour and breast tumour to tamoxifen. Subsequent surgery in the form of right mastectomy and axillary node clearance has led to this lady remaining disease free seven years following her surgery.

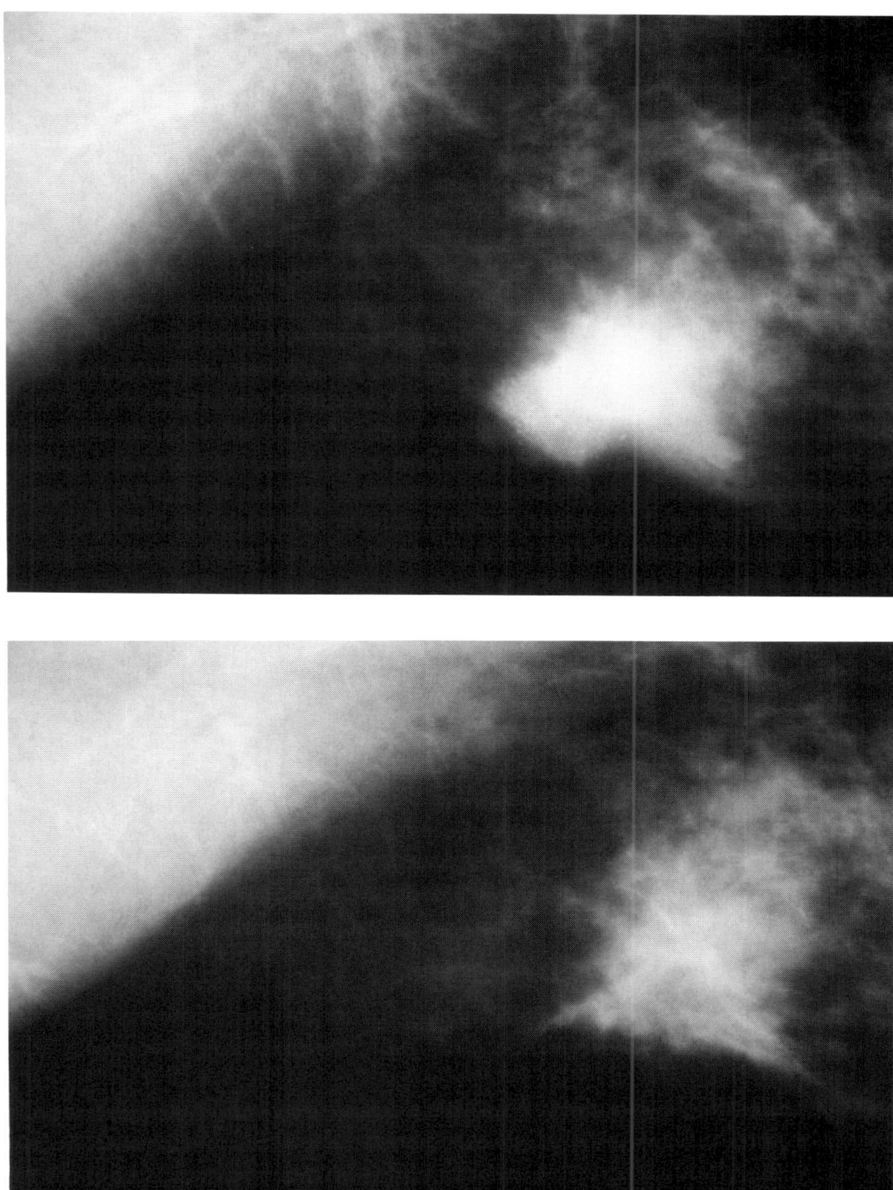

Fig. 4. (a) Large carcinoma of the upper outer quadrant of the breast with microcalcification within the tumour but not in the surrounding breast tissue, which (b) responded to chemotherapy with a partial response and subsequently underwent wide local excision and axillary node clearance followed by radiotherapy. Mammographic assessment is, however, difficult and ultrasound assessment provides a clear guide to response.

cal evidence of disease prior to surgery and a proportion of these patients will have a complete pathological response with no detectable disease in the surgical specimen. A partial response reflects a reduction of radiological and clinical size by more than 50% in more than one diameter. Stable disease (a <25% increase in two diameters or less than 50% decrease) and progressive disease (a >25% increase in size) should lead to change in therapy after three months. Radiological assessment of tumour size at present is by mammography or ultrasound [9]. Pre-treatment mammograms are required and should be repeated at three and six months as on occasion, when the oedema round the tumour settles, microcalcification outside the tumour becomes apparent (Fig. 4) [8,9]. Microcalcification is not visible on ultrasound. New methods of assessment such as magnetic resonance imaging and positron emission tomography (PET) remain purely for research at the present time, though the use of dynamic MRI to assess not only tumour size but vessel count/angiogenesis through therapy is one of the more interesting future possibilities [16]. Radiological assessment of tumour response in most studies, however, has been by mammography [1,3,8], despite the excellent data from the Edinburgh group suggesting that ultrasound is currently the best option [9]. Of 63 patients treated with neoadjuvant therapy whose tumour volume was subsequently measured at operation by a pathologist, ultrasound correlated best with pathological size measurement and correctly assessed response in 90% of women (compared to only 60% with mammography) [9].

A number of centres have different policy regimes after three months of treatment. If a tumour has not decreased in size some opt for mastectomy as non-responding tumours do badly and are usually unsuitable for breast conservation [6,10]. Other units would change to a different chemotherapy regimen. For tumours which have responded and are >1 cm in size most units would continue chemotherapy to attempt to obtain a complete response. In these cases some form of localisation is required prior to surgery [10]. It is clear that in the presence of progression at three months or stable disease, it is important to give consideration to change of therapy, as few responses are seen in the tumour after this time.

Other assessment of response

Of interest is the possibility that "change" in the biological parameters of a tumour would predict for response. Whilst this is currently not possible in routine practice it is a potentially important area of research. In particular, if we could predict which patients would remain node positive after chemotherapy despite good response in the primary tumour, different chemotherapy regimens might be adopted after three months. For instance, the presence of node positivity after neoadjuvant anthracycline regimens might lead to the use of adjuvant taxanes postoperatively.

Surgery

Local unit policy should guide whether non-responders receive their definite surgical procedure or are given alternative chemotherapy at three months. To achieve clear margins with responders skin tattooing should be performed at presentation after three months and chemotherapy should be continued to aim for a complete clinical response [1,10]. For those patients in whom the tumour had surrounding localised microcalcification pre-treatment, accurate localisation and specimen radiology may help to achieve clear margins. When localised microcalcification is seen on the original mammograms, specimen radiology should be used to ensure the whole lesion has been removed [10]. Some surgeons also advocate the use of frozen section histology to ensure margins are clear of tumour but this technique is notoriously unreliable compared to paraffin sections. We prefer to await final paraffin histology. Failure to achieve clear resection margins indicates a need for mastectomy.

Local recurrence

Surgery after chemotherapy is often difficult. Especially in non-responding tumours, the breast is frequently well vascularised whilst regression of axillary lymph nodes may be associated with fibrosis in the axilla, which makes dissection difficult. Care must be taken to ensure clear margins at wide local excision or mastectomy. Failure to clear margins of tumour is generally associated with a higher local recurrence rate. In addition, early studies suggested surgery after primary chemotherapy may be associated with a higher incidence of margin involvement [8], although this has not been subsequently borne out [3,6].

Zurrida et al. found local relapse after surgery was largely predicted by lack of response to primary chemotherapy [10]. Large tumours (greater than 3 cm in size) had a relapse of 22% compared to 5% in smaller tumours. Nodal involvement after surgery was also a marker for local relapse [10]. Jacquillat et al. found that tumour grade, size and tumour response were significant independent variables in predicting relapse after chemotherapy [17].

The timing of radiotherapy is another contentious issue: some studies have used it preoperatively but conventionally it is given postoperatively [18]. Colleoni reported that chemotherapy, then radiotherapy followed by surgery led to significantly increased postoperative complications. Relapse rates after short-term follow-up suggest a 2% local relapse rate/year [1,3,17-20], which is about double the normal local relapse rates after breast conservation (Table 1). However, nearly all women who relapse locally will have distant disease and will require systemic treatment. Thus the type of local surgery adopted does not appear to influence the overall prognosis.

Table 1. Relapse rates after primary chemotherapy

No. of patients	Breast relapse (%)		Distant relapse (%)		Follow-up (months)	Reference
83	2	(2%)	11	(13%)	12	[1]
192	20	(10%)	26	(14%)	62	[17]
126	2	(2%)	12	(10%)	30	[19]
158	11	(7%)	38	(24%)	38	[18]
50	2	(4%)	4	(6%)	15	[3]
97	10	(10%)	27	(28%)	36	[20]

Surgical morbidity and prognostic factors post-surgery

Little has been published on surgical complications after primary medical therapy [21-23]. Results from a prospective randomised trial in Edinburgh [21] found no increased morbidity in patients undergoing neoadjuvant therapy.

Studies suggest there is no increased incidence of morbidity postoperatively [21-23] and although nodal involvement is decreased there is still on average nodal metastasis in 50% of cases [1,2,8,10]. The optimum treatment of patients with such a poor prognosis is unclear and requires a randomised trial to determine whether further (different) chemotherapy is valuable. In addition, there is mounting evidence that node positivity predicts overall for poor survival [33].

New therapeutic approaches

Even the most optimistic oncologist must recognise the need to rethink breast cancer treatments in light of the apparent failure of high-dose chemotherapy to affect patient survival. Higher doses of chemotherapy alone are unlikely to succeed and novel therapeutic approaches are required.

The HER2 (c-erbB2) oncogene is amplified in around 20% of breast cancers and its presence confers resistance to antioestrogens [24]. A humanised murine monoclonal antibody to c-erbB2 has been developed which is called Trastuzumab [25,26]. In a prospective randomised controlled trial of chemotherapy given with or without Trastuzumab to 461 women with metastatic breast cancer, the addition of Trastuzumab significantly improved survival [27].

The identification that the c-erbB2 oncogene predicts for a poorer prognosis after primary medical therapy [7] and the potential benefit of Trastuzumab in c-erbB2-positive metastatic cancer suggests that a trial of primary medical therapy with or without Trastuzumab is warranted in c-erbB2 expressing breast cancers. Individualisation of neoadjuvant therapy is an exciting prospect which requires exploration in a research setting.

Other growth factor receptors (e.g. epidermal growth factor receptor) can now be targeted by drugs (e.g. ZD1839) and trials of primary chemotherapy with or without such drugs may provide a novel test-bed of such therapy [28].

Angiogenesis plays a critical role in tumour growth and metastasis. Continual formation of new capillaries is necessary for tumour growth and survival and in the absence of angiogenesis tumour growth cannot occur [29]. Phase I/II trials of antiangiogenic therapy are now being conducted in an attempt to target endothelial cells in tumours [30]. The use of an antiangiogenic drug in combination with chemotherapy may not only increase response rates but provide a suitable maintenance therapy after chemotherapy has ceased.

In this situation patients undergoing primary medical therapy provide an interesting clinical model to study the response of the endothelium to chemotherapy and antiangiogenic therapy and identification of novel endothelial markers of response such as serum VCAM/E selectin may enable assessment of response to therapy [31].

Conclusion

Primary medical therapy remains an important modality for the surgeon to be aware of. It is a potentially exciting area of research to elucidate tumour biology and response *in vivo*. Randomised clinical trials have shown no detrimental effect of neoadjuvant chemotherapy; there is thus the potential to combine neoadjuvant chemotherapy with or without other novel agents in further clinical trials.

References

1   Bonadonna G, Veronesi U, Brambilla C et al. Primary chemotherapy to avoid mastectomy in tumours with diameters of three centimeters or more. J Natl Cancer Inst 1990; 82(19): 1539-45

2   Fisher B, Brown A, Mamounas E et al. Effect of preoperative chemotherapy on local-regional disease in women with operable breast cancer: findings from National Surgical Adjuvant Breast and Bowel Project B-18. J Clin Oncol 1997; 15(7): 2483-93

3   Smith IE, Walsh G, Jones A et al. High complete remission rates with primary neoadjuvant infusional chemotherapy for large early breast cancer. J Clin Oncol 1995; 13(2): 424-9

4   Scholl SM, Fourquet A, Asselain B et al. Neoadjuvant versus adjuvant chemotherapy in premenopausal patients with tumours too large for breast conserving surgery: preliminary results of a randomised trial. Eur J Cancer 1994; 30A: 645-52

5   Mauriac L, Durand M, Avril A, Dilhuydy JM. Effects of primary chemotherapy in conservative treatment of breast cancer patients with operable tumours larger than 3 cm. Ann Oncol 1991; 2: 347-54

6   Anderson EDC, Forrest APM, Hawkins RA, Anderson TJ, Leonard RCF, Chetty U. Primary systemic therapy for operable breast cancer. Br J Cancer 1991; 63: 561-6

7   MacGrogan G, Mauriac L, Durand M et al. Primary chemotherapy in breast invasive carcinoma: predictive value of the immunohistochemical detection of hormonal receptors, p53, c-erbB-2, MiB1, pS2 and GST. Br J Cancer 1996; 74: 1458-65

8   Powles TJ, Hickish TF, Makris A et al. Randomized trial of chemoendocrine therapy started before or after surgery for treatment of primary breast cancer. J Clin Oncol 1995; 13(3): 547-52

9   Farouli P, Walsh JS, Anderson TJ, Chetty U. Ultrasound as a method of measuring breast tumour size and monitoring response to primary systemic treatment. Br J Surg 1994; 81: 223-5

10   Zurrida S, Greco M, Veronesi U. Surgical pitfalls after pre-operative chemotherapy in large size breast cancer. Eur J Surg Oncol 1994; 20: 641-3

11   Hawkins RA, Tesdale AL, Anderson EDC et al. Does the oestrogen receptor concentration of breast cancer change during systemic therapy. Br J Cancer 1990; 61: 877-80

12   Mansi J, Smith I, Walsh G et al. Primary medical therapy for operable breast cancer. Eur J Cancer Clin Oncol 1989; 25(11): 1623-7

13   Horobin JM, Preece PE, Dewar JA et al. 5-12 year follow up of elderly patients with localised breast cancer treated whose sole primary treatment was tamoxifen. Br J Surg 1991; 78: 213

14   Isola JJ, Helin HJ, Helle MJ et al. Evaluation of cell proliferation in breast carcinoma: comparison of Ki67 in immunohistological study with DNA flow cytometric analysis and mitotic count. Cancer 1990; 65: 1180-4

15   Ravdin PM, Green S, Albain KS et al. Initial report of the SWOG biological correlative study of cerbb2 expression as a predictor of outcome in a trial comparing adjuvant CAFT with Tamoxifen (T). Proc ASCO 1988; 7: A374

16   Gilties R, Guinebetiere JM, Toussant O. Locally advanced breast cancer: Contrast enhanced subtraction MR imaging of response to preoperative chemotherapy. Radiology 1994; 191: 633-8

17   Jacquillat C, Weil M, Ballet F et al. Results of neoadjuvant chemotherapy and radiation therapy in the breast conserving treatment of 250 patients with all stages of infiltrative breast cancer. Cancer 1990; 66: 119-29

18   Calais G, Berger C, Descamps P et al. Conservative treatment feasibility with induction chemotherapy, surgery and radiotherapy for patients with breast carcinoma larger than 3 cm. Cancer 1994; 74: 1283-3

19   Belambaogo E, Feillel V, Challet P et al. Neoadjuvant chemotherapy in 126 operable breast cancers. Eur J Cancer 1992; 28A: 286-90

20   Bramley MD, Harake J, Boggis CRM, Howell A, Bundred NJ. Neoadjuvant chemotherapy for primary breast cancer – how many breasts are saved? Eur J Cancer 1998; 34(5): S53

21   Forouhi P, Dixon JM, Leonard RCF, Chetty U. Prospective randomised study of surgical morbidity following primary systemic therapy for breast cancer. Br J Surg 1995; 82: 79-82

22   Darforth DN, Lippman ME, McDonald H et al. Effect of preoperative chemotherapy on mastectomy for locally advanced breast cancer. Ann Surg 1990; 56: 6-11

23   Broadwater JR, Edwards MJ, Kuglen C, Hortobagyi GN, Aves FC, Balch CM. Mastectomy following preoperative chemotherapy: strict operative criteria control operative morbidity. Ann Surg 1991; 213: 126-9

24   Slamon DJ, Clark GM, Wong SG et al. Human breast cancer: correlation of relapse and survival with amplification of the Her2/neu oncogene. Science 1987; 235: 177-82

25   Carter P, Goman CM, Presta L et al. Humanisation of an anti-p185 HER2 antibody for human cancer therapy. Proc Natl Acad Sci USA 1992; 89: 4285-9

26   Cobleigh MA, Vogel CL, Tripatry NJ et al. Efficacy and safety of Herceptin™ as a single agent in 222 women with HER2 overexpression who relapsed following chemotherapy for metastatic breast cancer. Proc ASCO 1998; 17: A376

27   Slamon D, Leyland-Jones B, Shak S et al. Addition of Herceptin to first line chemotherapy for HER2 overexpressing metastatic breast cancer (HER2 HMBC) markedly increases anticancer activity a randomised, multinational controlled phase III trial. Proc ASCO 1998; 17: A377

28 Woodburn JR, Morris CQ, Kelly H, Laight A. EGF receptor tyrosine kinase inhibitors as anti-cancer agents – pre-clinical and early clinical profile of ZD1839. Cell Mol Biol (Letters) 1998; 5: 348-9
29 Fidler IJ, Ellis LM. The implications of angiogenesis for the biology and therapy of cancer metastasis. Cell 1994; 79: 185-8
30 Bicknell R, Harris AL. Novel growth regulatory factors and tumour angiogenesis. Eur J Cancer 1991; 27: 781-4
31 Byrne GJ, Blann AD, Venizelos V, Iddon J, Howell A, Bundred NJ. Serum VCAM and ESEL are endothelial markers for angiogenesis in early and advanced breast cancer. Eur J Surg Oncol 1997; 23: 372
32 Colleoni M, Nole F, Minchella I et al. Pre-operative chemotherapy and radiotherapy in breast cancer. Eur J Cancer 1998; 34(5): 641-5
33 Touboul E, Lefranc J, Blondon J et al. Primary chemotherapy and preoperative irradiation for patients with stage II larger than 3 cm or locally advanced non-inflammatory breast cancer. Radiol Oncol 1997; 42: 219-29

ESO Scientific Updates, Vol. 4
Primary Medical Therapy for Breast Cancer
A. Howell and M. Dowsett, editors
© 1999 Elsevier Science B.V. All rights reserved

Biological Markers and Changes Induced in their Profiles Following Primary Chemotherapy: Relevance for Short- and Long-Term Clinical Outcome

Maria Grazia Daidone[1], Silvia Veneroni[1], Elvira Benini[1], Gorana Tomasic[3], Danila Coradini[1], Cristina Brambilla[2], Laura Ferrari[2] and Rosella Silvestrini[1]

1   Department of Experimental Oncology, Unit 10
2   Department of Medical Oncology
3   Division of Anatomical Pathology, Istituto Nazionale per lo Studio e la Cura dei Tumori, Milan, Italy

Introduction

An objective of translational studies on human tumours has been the search for biomarkers to use as a complement to clinicopathological staging in order to identify patients destined to relapse or progression independent of treatment, and to predict which patients are likely to respond or develop resistance to a specific treatment [1]. The contribution of factors related to functional aspects specific to some cancers (such as hormone and growth factor receptors) or common to all tumour types (such as cell proliferation, invasiveness or angiogenesis markers, DNA ploidy and alterations or dysregulation of oncogenes and tumour-suppressor genes) has been defined for the identification of patients at high risk of relapse (who need aggressive systemic treatments) and of patients with an indolent disease course (who are potentially curable by local-regional treatment alone) [2].

Recently, the interest of investigators involved in translational studies in breast cancer has been focused on the evaluation of the role of biomarkers as indicators of response to chemical and physical treatments [3]. In addition to validation of the predictive role of steroid receptors as indicators of endocrine susceptibility, preliminary studies have suggested a potential relevance for cell proliferation [4-7], HER2/neu expression [8-10] and, more recently, for p53 [11,12] and bax [13] as predictors of response to systemic chemotherapy.

Address for correspondence: M.G. Daidone, Department of Experimental Oncology - Unit 10, Istituto Nazionale Tumori, Via Venezian 1, 20133 Milan, Italy. Tel.: +39-02-2390238, fax: +39-02-2364366, e-mail: daidone@istitutotumori.mi.it

However, most of these studies have been retrospectively performed in adjuvant settings in which the advantage of a long-term follow-up was counterbalanced by a marked heterogeneity in the technical procedures (type and time of fixation, storage conditions) used to process and store archival specimens. More recently, the determination of biomarkers has been prospectively planned within the context of adjuvant and neoadjuvant treatment protocols, in which the evaluation of utility of biological information represented a secondary objective of the clinical study. Although such studies have not been specifically designed to test marker predictiveness, it is likely that they will improve the quality of information on the predictive accuracy of tumour markers and provide a definite evaluation of their clinical utility.

Among the different approaches used in translational studies, neoadjuvant chemotherapy could represent an ideal model to evaluate the clinical impact of biological investigations, to analyse the predictiveness of biological variables in relation to different clinical endpoints, and to monitor, both at the cellular and molecular level, treatment effect by sequential determination of biomarkers within a single tumour, in the presence of only intralesional heterogeneity [14].

Overview of published results

In the last four years, a number of studies have been published by independent groups which analysed the role of biological markers in several different protocols of primary chemotherapy involving about 1800 women with operable and locally advanced breast cancer [11,15-40]. Different biological aspects were investigated including cell proliferation, hormone and growth factor receptors, differentiation, gross or specific genomic alterations or dysfunctions, markers related to apoptosis, invasion and angiogenesis, and markers concurring to determine resistance to specific antineoplastic agents (Table 1). Biomarkers were determined before starting primary treatment, at the time of initial diagnosis, and in some studies the determinations were repeated on tumour material taken at surgery or during the early stages of treatment [15-28]. The latter approach, in which information for biological studies should be obtained with the tumour remaining *in vivo*, implied a preliminary assessment of feasibility and reliability on tumour specimens taken by non-traumatic methods, such as fine needle aspiration [41,42].

Overall, significant changes after treatment were mainly observed in markers of proliferation, differentiation, apoptosis and multidrug resistance. They generally consisted of a reduction in the proliferative activity and in the expression of proliferation markers (evaluated by ^{3}H-thymidine labelling index [TLI], flow-cytometric S-phase fraction [FCM-S] and mitotic activity index [MAI], and by Ki67/Mib1, respectively) [15,16,18,19,22,23,25,27], of an enhancement in bcl-2 expression [18,22-24], and of an acquired or increased mdr1 gene expression [20]. Conversely, steroid receptors and gross or specific genomic alterations appeared to be changed minimally or not at all [15,16,24,25].

Table 1. Summary of studies published from 1995 to 1998 evaluating biological markers in primary chemotherapy trials for breast cancer

1st Author (reference)	Stage (# cases)	Treatment	Investigated variables	Monitoring	Clinical relevance
Bottini [15]	II_A-III_B (99)	Dx or CMF(+ Tam if ER+)→Surgery	Ki67, ER & PgR*, HER2*	↓ Ki67 No change for ER, PgR, HER2	
Daidone [16]	II_A-B (123)	CMF, FAC, FEC, FNC, Dx	TLI, FCM-S, ER, PgR, ploidy, p53*, bcl-2	Changes for TLI and FCM-S; minimal changes for ER, PgR, ploidy, p53, bcl-2	
Ellis [17]	II_A-B (27)	FEC, EC	Ki67, AI, bcl-2	↑ AI No change for Ki67, bcl-2	
Baldini [18]	III_A-B (96)	FEC+GM-CSF →Surgery→FEC/CMF	TLI, IGF-1R, bcl-2	↓ TLI and IGF-1R ↑ bcl-2	OCR related only to high pre-CT TLI
Briffod [19]	II_A-B (94)	AVCMF or FEC →Surgery	FCM-S, ploidy, HG	Changes for FCM-S, ploidy, HG	OCR related to high pre-CT HG and FCM-S, and to DNA and cytomorphological changes
Chevillard [20]	II_A-III_B (87)	FAC, FTC	FCM-S, ER, PgR, ploidy, MDR1**, Pgp*	Acquired or ↑ MDR1gene expression Acquired Pgp expression	OCR related to pre-CT high FCM-S, MDR1⁻ and to constant MDR1⁻ after the 1st CT cycle
Cocconi [21]	II_A-B (NS)	CMF, CMFEV →Surgery	Ki67, ER & PgR*, p53*	Changes	CR related to ↓ ER and PgR and to ↑ Ki67

Table 1. Summary of studies published from 1995 to 1998 evaluating biological markers in primary chemotherapy trials for breast cancer (contd.)

1st Author (reference)	Stage (# cases)	Treatment	Investigated variables	Monitoring	Clinical relevance
Collecchi [22]	III$_{A-B}$ (70)	FEC→Surgery→ FEC/CMF	TLI, bcl-2	Changes for TLI, ↑ bcl-2	OCR related only to high pre-CT TLI DFS related only to low post-CT TLI
Ellis [23]	II$_{A-B}$ (40)	FEC→Surgery	Ki67, ER**, AI, bcl-2	↓ Ki67, ER, AI ↑ bcl-2	CR unrelated to pre-CT values or changes of biomarkers; PR related to ↓ AI
Frassoldati [24]	III$_{A-B}$ (29)	Not specified	HG, Ki67, PCNA, ER & PgR*, EGFR, p53*, AI, bcl-2, Pgp*	↑ PCNA, EGFR, AI, bcl-2, Pgp No change for HG, Ki67, ER, PgR, p53	OCR related to ↓ ER No response related to ↑ PCNA and EGFR
Honkoop [25,26]	III$_{A-B}$ (42)	Not specified	Ki67, MAI, ploidy, CD31, p53*, Pgp*	↓ MAI and CD31 No consistent changes for Ki67, ploidy, p53, Pgp	OCR unrelated to patho-biological features Unfavourable outcome related to high post-CT Ki67 and to Pgp and p53 co-expression
Moll [27]	III (61)	Not specified	HG, MI, p53*	Changes for MI and HG	OCR unrelated to pre-CT p53
Pierga [28]	II$_{A-B}$ (69)	FAC, FEC→Surgery	FCM-S, ER, PgR, ploidy, PAI-1, uPA	↓ PAI-1	OCR related only to high pre-CT FCM-S

Table 1. Summary of studies published from 1995 to 1998 evaluating biological markers in primary chemotherapy trials for breast cancer (contd.)

1st Author (reference)	Stage (# cases)	Treatment	Investigated variables	Monitoring	Clinical relevance
Aas [11]	III$_A$-B (63)	Dx	p53*,***		OCR related only to specific TP53 mutations OS related to specific TP53 mutations and protein expression
Akashi-Tanaka [29]	III$_A$-B (37)	Not specified	HG, MI		OCR & OS related to low HG and MI
Bonetti [30]	III$_A$-B,IV (76)	CMF, FAC or FEC	Ki67, ER*		OCR related to high Ki67 OS related to low Ki67 only in responsive patients
Bonetti [31]	III$_A$-B,IV (55)	CMF, FAC or FEC	Ki67, ER*, bcl-2, p53*		OCR related to low bcl-2 and ER⁻ OS not related to bcl-2
Bottini [32]	II$_A$-III$_B$ (76)	Dx or CMF(+ Tam if ER$^+$)→Surgery	Ki67, ER & PgR*		CR and PR related to ↓ Ki67 DFS related to no change or to ↓ Ki67
MacGrogan [33]	II$_A$-B (128)	Not specified	Mib1, ER & PgR*, pS2, p53, HER2*, GSTπ*		OCR related to ER⁻ and high pre-CT Mib1 OS, DFS, MFS related to HER2 overexpression

Table 1. Summary of studies published from 1995 to 1998 evaluating biological markers in primary chemotherapy trials for breast cancer (contd.)

1st Author (reference)	Stage (# cases)	Treatment	Investigated variables	Monitoring	Clinical relevance
Makris [34]	NS (57)	MMT	p53*		OCR unrelated to p53
Paulsen [36]	III$_{A-B}$ (63)	Dx	MVD		OCR unrelated to MVD
Remvikos [37]	II$_{A-B}$ (127)	FAC→Surgery or RT	HG, FCM-S, ER, PgR		MFS and OS related only to low pre-CT FCM-S
Rozan [38]	II$_{A-B}$ (167)	FAC→Surgery	HG, FCM-S, Mib1, p53, HER2*		CR related only to high pre-CT HG and FCM-S
Wang [39]	NS (33)	AC	p53*, MDR1**, Pgp*		Response to Dx related only to Pgp
Willsher [40]	III$_{A-B}$ (50)	MMM→Surgery	Mib1, HER2*		OCR related only to pre-CT HER2-

List of abbreviations

AI, apoptotic index
EGFR, epidermal growth factor receptor
FCM-S, flow-cytometric S-phase cell fraction
GSTπ, glutathione-S-transferase π
HG, histological grading
IGF-1R, insulin-like growth factor-1 receptor
MAI, mitotic activity index
MDR, multi-drug resistance
MVD, microvessel density
NS, not specified
PAI-1, plasminogen activator inhibitor-1
PCNA, proliferating cell nuclear antigen
Pgp, P-glycoprotein
Pre-CT, post-CT, before or after primary chemotherapy treatment
TLI, ^{3}H-thymidine labelling index
uPA, urokinase plasminogen activator

Treatments

AC, doxorubicin, cyclophosphamide; AVCMF, doxorubicin, vincristine, cyclophosphamide, methotrexate, 5-fluorouracil; CMF, cyclophosphamide, methotrexate, 5-fluorouracil; CMFEV, cyclophosphamide, methotrexate, 5-fluorouracil, epirubicin, vincristine; Dx, doxorubicin; EC, epirubicin, cyclophosphamide; FAC, 5-fluorouracil, doxorubicin, cyclophosphamide; FEC, 5-fluorouracil, epirubicin, cyclophosphamide; FNC, 5-fluorouracil, mitoxantrone, cyclophosphamide; FTC, 5-fluorouracil, thiotepa, cyclophosphamide; GM-CSF, granulocyte-macrophage colony stimulating factor; MMM, mitoxantrone, methotrexate, mitomycin; MMT, mitoxantrone, methotrexate, tamoxifen.

Methodological approaches

*, determined by immunohisto- or cytochemistry; **, determined by RT-PCR (reverse transcriptase-polymerase chain reaction); ***, determined by CGDE (constant denaturant gel electrophoresis).

Clinical endpoints

CR, complete response; DFS, disease-free survival; MFS, metastasis-free survival; OCR, objective clinical response; OS, overall survival; PR, partial remission.

Tumour shrinkage proved to be less frequent in patients presenting before treatment with slowly proliferating tumours [18-22,28,30,33,38], steroid receptor positivity [21,24,31,33], specific TP53 mutations [11] or exhibiting, after few treatment courses, changes in the expression of mdr markers [20]. A favourable long-term clinical outcome was generally, although not universally, observed for patients with indolent tumours post-treatment, i.e. tumours that were slowly proliferating [22,26,29,30,32], with wild-type TP53 [11], and weakly or not expressing p53 or HER2 [11,26,33].

In this chapter we present our experience with biological characterisation including the evaluation of proliferation indices, DNA ploidy, hormone receptors, proliferation and apoptosis-related markers within a clinical protocol of primary chemotherapy, and report the analysis of changes in biomarkers following treatment and the association of these changes with clinical outcome.

Biological markers and primary chemotherapy: Experience at the Istituto Nazionale Tumori of Milan

Case series

At the Istituto Nazionale Tumori of Milan, during the period January 1988 to October 1990, a prospective non-randomised study of primary chemotherapy was conducted in which 231 women with histologically diagnosed breast tumours larger than 3 cm were enrolled [43]. Consecutive groups of patients received different drug regimens consisting of three or four cycles of cyclophosphamide, methotrexate and 5-fluorouracil (CMF) or 5-fluorouracil, adriamycin and cyclophosphamide (FAC), three cycles of 5-fluorouracil, cyclophosphamide plus epirubicin (FEC) or novantrone (FNC), or three cycles of adriamycin. Surgery (modified mastectomy or quadrantectomy) was planned within three weeks of the last primary chemotherapy dose. As an ancillary part of the clinical study, a panel of biological markers which included S-phase fraction indicators evaluated by autoradiography as TLI [44] and by flow cytometry [45], distribution of cells in the cell cycle, DNA ploidy [45], and steroid hormone receptors evaluated by DCC [46], was prospectively determined before starting treatment, at the time of diagnosis on incisional biopsy, and the determinations were repeated at the end of primary chemotherapy, at the time of radical surgery [16]. Successively the biological information was integrated with determination of the immunohistochemical expression of p53 [47], bcl-2 [48] and bax [49]. The availability of the biological information depended on the priority given to the determination of different markers (hormone receptors first, followed by TLI and DNA content) owing to the relatively small biopsy samples [16], on the gross disappearance of tumour material at surgery, or on the occurrence of progressive disease during chemotherapy (in 3% of the cases), which prevented or affected the timing of surgery. In addition, determination of p53, bcl-2 and bax was dependent on the availability of adequate tumour material from paraffin-embedded specimens used for the routine determination of TLI. In this series of cases we analysed the changes induced by primary chemotherapy in proliferation rate, nuclear DNA content and hormone receptor status, and in the expression of p53, bcl-2 and bax proteins, and we assessed the predictive role of pre-treatment and post-treatment biological markers in relation to the different clinical endpoints.

Changes in biological markers after primary chemotherapy

Overall, after three or four cycles of primary chemotherapy there was a decrease in the tumour's proliferative activity, which was of a similar degree for both TLI and FCM-S, and in the fraction of progesterone receptor-positive (PgR+) and aneuploid tumours (Table 2). Conversely, on the whole the frequency of tumours with detectable oestrogen receptors (ER) or immunoreactive for p53, bcl-2 and bax expression was similar before and after treatment. When the pattern of change was analysed in individual tumours, variations in the proliferative indices mainly consisted of a decrease for rapidly proliferating tumours (in 44% or 54% of the cases when TLI or FCM-S was considered), whereas an increase or no change was more frequently observed for slowly proliferating tumours. Such changes were largely independent of the treatment regimen administered. Conversely, a higher accumulation of cells in the G2M phases was detected by FCM after anthracycline-containing regimens than after CMF [16], which is in agreement with the mechanism of action of doxorubicin and related drugs and with previously published results [50].

Hormone receptors and DNA ploidy showed only minimal changes, since the concordance between pre- and post-treatment ER and PgR status and DNA content was 79%, 75% and 74%, respectively, regardless of the treatment given. Specific changes (Table 2) consisted of appearance of ER in 30% of pre-treatment ER− tumours, disappearance of PgR in about 40% of PgR− tumours, and loss of aneuploid clones in 30% of initially aneuploid tumours.

As regards markers that control apoptosis either negatively, such as bcl-2, or positively, such as bax [51], bcl-2 expression was unaffected in about 80% of cases, whereas bax expression remained virtually unaltered in tumours not or weakly expressing the marker but decreased in 60% of those overexpressing it (Table 2). p53 expression was similar before and after treatment in about 75% of the cases; in particular, p53 expression remained unchanged in 90% of p53-negative tumours and significantly decreased in 60% of initially overexpressing tumours, thus suggesting a possible disappearance of p53-positive subpopulations. When single-strand conformation polymorphism analysis for p53 was performed in 11 of these cases, chemotherapy treatment did not seem to induce band shifts in the five negative cases nor to modify those present in the six positive cases, in accordance with what has been observed in other tumour types [52].

In conclusion, primary chemotherapy seems to affect proliferation indices, with changes that are related to pre-treatment biological characteristics, and to induce cell accumulation in the G2M phases when anthracyclines are in-

Table 2. Biological markers determined before and after primary chemotherapy (CT)

	Pre-CT	Post-CT	Peculiar changes following treatment
Proliferative activity			
TLI (median, %)	4.4	3.6	
% high TLI cases	69	53	Reduction in 44% of pre-CT high TLI cases (p < 0.0001)
FCM-S (median, %)	7.2	4.9	
% high FCM-S cases	66	52	Reduction in 54% of pre-CT high FCM-S cases (p < 0.0001)
Hormone receptors			
% ER⁻cases	38	40	ER detectable in 30% of pre-CT ER⁻ tumours
% PgR⁻ cases	51	70	Loss of PgR in 38% of pre-CT PgR$^+$
DNA content			
% aneuploid cases	79	62	Loss of aneuploidy in 30% of pre-CT aneuploid cases
p53 expression			
% p53$^+$ cases	34	29	Reduced expression in 38% of pre-CT p53$^+$ cases (p = 0.01)
bcl-2 expression			
% bcl-2⁻ cases	59	65	Unrelated to basic expression
bax expression			
% bax$^+$ cases	34	31	Reduced expression in 60% of pre-CT bax$^+$ cases (p = 0.01)

cluded in the treatment regimen. In addition, it seems to reduce the fraction of p53 and bax-positive cells and PgR content, whereas it induces minor or no changes in ploidy, steroid receptors and bcl-2 expression. The pattern of significant or minimal changes observed for proliferation markers, DNA content, hormone receptor status and p53 expression, and the specific cell cycle perturbations following anthracycline-containing regimens are consistent with results reported by other studies [15,17-19,22-25,50], some of which differ from ours in terms of clinical (type of intercurrent treatment and timing of sequential biopsies) and methodological conditions (tumour specimens obtained by fine needle aspiration, different approaches used to evaluate the same biological feature). Moreover, we confirmed in a successive study conducted at our Institute on a series of 319 cases undergoing primary chemotherapy with single-agent anthracycline [53] in which only fine needle aspirates were available at the time of initial diagnosis, the modulation of cells in FCM-S, the accumulation of cells in the G_2M phase and the minimal variations in DNA content. In partial disagreement with results reported by other authors [18,22-24], we observed a minor involvement of bcl-2 expression when monitoring the biological response to primary chemotherapy at the cellular level. Such a finding is probably due to the long interval between biopsy and surgery in our experimental set-up, which might be inadequate to detect changes in apoptosis-related markers.

Association between biological markers and clinical outcome

Tumour shrinkage

When we analysed objective clinical response as a function of biological variables, pre-treatment values and their changes were considered. Significant predictors of tumour reduction were only PgR status (p = 0.03) and p53 expression (p = 0.003), even though their predictive value was relatively weak (Table 3). In fact, 86% of patients with tumours that were PgR negative or did not express p53 achieved clinical response, which was also obtained by about two thirds of patients whose tumours showed the opposite biological profile. The predictiveness of p53 or PgR expression for tumour shrinkage was more evident in subsets given anthracycline-containing regimens (p = 0.048) or in tumours smaller than 5 cm (p = 0.06), respectively. None of the other markers related to proliferation or to apoptosis, or their changes detected after treatment, provided significant information on clinical response, and the results were similar even when analysed within the different chemotherapy regimens.

Taken together, these findings represent a confirmation of preliminary results obtained in an initial subset of cases [43], and provide further support to the concept of p53 alterations as determinants of drug resistance, which already emerged in different tumour types and especially in breast cancer following anthracycline-containing regimens [11,12,54,55]. However, the achievement of clinical response in about 80% of the cases entering this clinical protocol [43,53] could in part limit the clinical utility of biological markers to predict tumour shrinkage.

Table 3. Objective clinical response to primary chemotherapy by pre-treatment values of biological markers as a function of treatment

	CMF		Anthracycline-containing regimens	
	No. of cases	PR ≥ 50%*	No. of cases	PR ≥ 50%
Proliferative activity				
Low TLI	11	73	40	85
High TLI	36	67	77	79
Hormone receptors				
ER$^+$	36	64	39	82
ER$^-$	7	86	41	83
PgR$^+$	32	62	27	74
PgR$^-$	11	82	53	87
DNA content				
Diploid	8	62	21	95
Aneuploid	36	69	71	83
p53 expression				
p53$^-$	20	80	70	89
p53$^+$	16	62	30	70
bcl-2 expression				
bcl-2$^+$	15	53	31	84
bcl-2$^-$	12	75	55	87
bax expression				
bax$^-$	12	58	42	86
bax$^+$	5	60	23	83

* Partial response ≥50%, i.e., tumour shrinkage greater than 50% compared to inital measurements

Relapse-free survival

Following surgery, the clinical protocol activated at the Istituto Nazionale Tumori of Milan required adjuvant postoperative treatment for all women with positive lymph nodes (N^+) as well as for those with negative nodes (N^-) but at high risk because their tumours were oestrogen receptor negative (ER^-) [43,53]. In responding patients, depending on the number of cycles administered during primary chemotherapy, two or three courses of the same combination were planned as adjuvant postoperative treatment, with the exception of women given primary adriamycin alone, who were treated after surgery with three cycles of CMF. For patients that were not responsive to primary chemotherapy a non-cross-resistant regimen was planned. Adjuvant chemotherapy was started 8-10 days after surgery and was delivered simultaneously with breast irradiation in patients subjected to breast conserving surgery, without discontinuation of any drug included in the combination [53].

The predictive value of pre- and post-treatment biological variables for relapse-free survival was initially analysed on the overall series of patients undergoing primary chemotherapy, regardless of the treatment administered following surgery. Pretreatment values of all the investigated variables were unrelated to clinical outcome at seven years. When post-treatment biological variables were considered, only hormone receptors predicted the occurrence of new disease manifestations, in particular ER, with a relapse rate about 1.5 times higher for patients presenting at surgery with ER^+ compared to ER^- tumours (57% vs 36%, p = 0.007). This was true even for patients receiving postoperative adjuvant treatment (Table 4), i.e., women presenting at surgery with N^+ or ER^-/N^- tumours (about 70% of the cases), for whom a trend in favour of a relation with clinical oucome emerged also for PgR (relapse rate 45% for PgR^- vs 64% for PgR^+). In this subset an exploratory subset analysis was carried out as a function of disease extent following primary treatment. For women presenting at surgery with ER^-/N^- or 1-3 N^+ tumours, which included the majority of the cases undergoing postoperative adjuvant treatment and could be considered as a subset with putatively chemoresponsive tumours, besides the long-term predictive role of ER or PgR, a trend in favour of a higher probability of 7-year relapse-free survival emerged for patients with rapidly proliferating, bcl-2-negative or bax-positive tumours (Table 4).

In this subset of patients a better identification of women with favourable outcome was provided by the combined consideration of apoptosis-related markers or of ER and TLI rather than by the four markers considered singly. In fact, the absence of ER in rapidly proliferating tumours was associated with an 80% probability of no relapse at seven years compared to the about 30% probability for patients with ER^+ tumours, regardless of their proliferative status (Fig. 1). An intermediate probability of relapse-free survival (50%) was observed for patients whose tumours were ER^- but slowly proliferating. If such results, which emerged or are emerging also in other adjuvant settings [7,56-58], are confirmed by a longer follow-up and validated by independent studies, the

Table 4. Seven-year clinical outcome by post-treatment values of biological markers in patients given postoperative adjuvant chemotherapy

	% Relapse-free survival		
	Overall	N^-/ER^-, 1-3N+	$>3N^+$
Proliferative activity			
Low TLI	39	42	35
High TLI	49	61	27
Hormone receptors			
ER^+	36*	40	31
ER^-	64*	67	45
PgR^+	36**	47	27
PgR^-	55**	59	42
DNA content			
Diploid	58	55	53
Aneuploid	49	62	24
p53 expression			
$p53^-$	49	56	35
$p53^+$	34	44	18
bcl-2 expression			
$bcl-2^+$	43	38	50
$bcl-2^-$	44	60	19
bax expression			
bax^-	41	46	33
bax^+	54	63	33

* $p = 0.0037$, ** $p = 0.07$

absence of steroid receptors and rapid proliferation should be considered as a biological profile predictive of treatment response, particularly when anti-metabolites are included in the regimens. However, such results are not common for all published translational studies in which information on cell proliferation and steroid receptors is available. Beside heterogeneity in the investigated case series and in the type and schedule of administered drugs, also differences in the technical approaches used to detect a single biological feature (e.g.

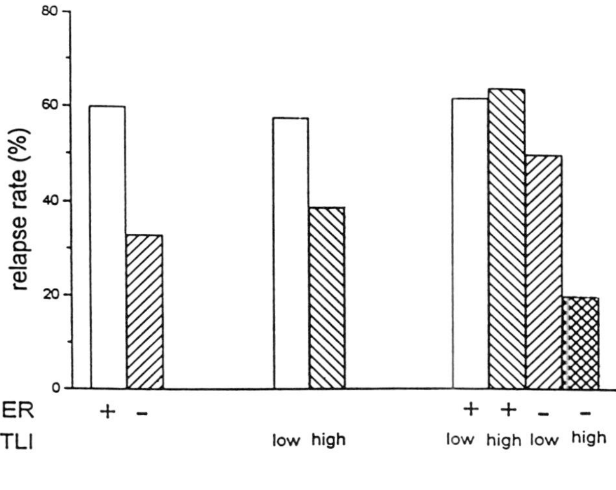

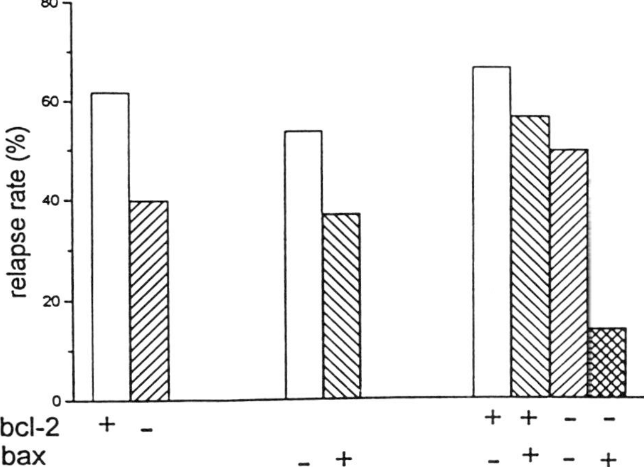

Fig. 1. Relapse rate as a function of post-treatment ER and TLI, bcl-2 and bax singly and in association in the subset of patients with ER⁻/N⁻ or 1-3 N⁺ tumours receiving postoperative adjuvant treatment.

S-phase fraction evaluated by TLI or FCM-S; hormone receptors detected by the dextran-coated charcoal technique or by immunohistochemistry), as well as in the markers evaluating different aspects of the same biological process (e.g. cell proliferation determined by TLI/FCM-S, Ki67 or PCNA) could account for some of the contrasting results [30, 37].

As regards markers influencing apoptosis, a weak or absent expression of the anti-apoptotic gene bcl-2 or the expression of the pro-apoptotic gene bax, which promote apoptosis and appear to be determinants of cellular response to genotoxic damage [51,59], are singly associated with a favourable outcome following chemotherapy (Table 4). Such a finding is reinforced by the significant association of the combined expression of bcl-2 and bax with relapse-free survival. In fact, patients with bcl-2-positive and bax-negative tumours, i.e. with both markers preventing apoptosis, had an about fourfold higher probability of relapse than patients whose tumours exhibited the opposite biological profile, i.e. the absence of bcl-2 and the presence of bax, which both favour the apoptotic programme (70% vs 15%) (Fig. 1). An intermediate relapse rate was observed for patients whose tumours expressed only one of the apoptosis-promoting factors. Such findings, which need to be confirmed by independent studies, are consistent with the hypothesis of an involvement of pro- and anti-apoptotic proteins in determining the fate of tumour cells exposed to anticancer agents [13, 31].

Owing to the small number of cases, only descriptive and qualitative data were reported for patients presenting at surgery with more than three positive axillary lymph nodes (Table 4). Overall, relapse-free survival was slightly superior for patients whose tumours exhibited features indicative of a low biological aggressiveness (i.e., low proliferation, absence of p53 expression, overexpression of bcl-2 and presence of only diploid clones) than for patients whose tumours exhibited the opposite biological profile. Also the small number of cases with biologically characterised tumours belonging to the subset of N^-, low-risk (i.e., ER^+) tumours precluded any meaningful analysis of clinical outcome as a function of biological markers in the subset of patients receiving no systemic adjuvant postoperative treatment.

Concluding remarks

The finding that biological markers determined before or after primary chemotherapy are different in terms of their predictiveness of long-term outcome following surgery should give significance to the biological profile of residual tumour cells after treatment and clinical relevance to post-treatment changes, even though they are minimal, such as those observed for steroid hormone receptors and apoptosis-related markers [16]. Our results suggest that clinical outcome following primary medical treatment is associated with the expression in surgical specimens of features indicative of biological aggressiveness but, possibly, even of susceptibility to drug effects, such as steroid receptor negativity [58], high proliferative activity [4], and markers favouring apoptosis [13,31,60]. Such an association is mainly evident in patients receiving postoperative adjuvant chemotherapy in whom the extent of nodal involvement, histologically assessed at surgery, was relatively limited. All these findings, however, are derived from a subset analysis and should thus be considered as hypothesis generating and requiring further validation.

Despite emerging evidence of the clinical relevance of the pathobiological profile of residual tumour cells after treatment, the most important constraint on the feasibility of the different biological determinations in a primary medical trial remains the reduction of viable tumour material after primary chemotherapy, which limits and possibly selects the fraction of cases eligible for translational studies. For this reason, which is likely to affect most of the studies in the neoadjuvant setting, our findings must be considered preliminary, although they are in keeping with previous results from our as well as other groups.

Primary chemotherapy appears to be and actually could be considered as an ideal model to investigate the predictive value of biological markers with respect to various clinical endpoints. However, the outcome of published translational studies in this area is quite controversial, and currently available data appear insufficient to derive statements on the clinical utility of biomarkers and, more importantly, recommend their use for the selection of different treatment options. A consensus should be reached on the results of translational studies within primary chemotherapy trials. In addition, several issues remain to be resolved before the outcome of a pathobiological characterisation could be translated to the clinical practice. These issues can be summarised as follows:

1. assessment of the adequate timing for post-treatment biopsy to detect alterations of biological markers which are specific as well as sensitive enough to parallel clinical outcome;
2. evaluation of the assessability of biological markers in post-treatment specimens, which is critical when treatment has been particularly effective at a cellular level and, consequently, definition of the clinical utility of a biological characterisation and setup of reliable approaches requiring minimal tumour specimens;
3. definition of the biological significance of residual tumour cells and of markers detected in these cells;
4. assessment of the consistency of the predictiveness of biomarkers for long-term clinical outcome.

Acknowledgements

Our work was supported by grants from the Italian Association for Cancer Research (AIRC), the Italian Research Council (CNR), and the Italian Ministry of Health.
We thank B. Canova for editorial assistance, and R. Motta, G. Abolafio and R. Erdas for their skillful technical collaboration.

References

1   Tumor Marker Expert Panel Members: Clinical practice guidelines for the use of tumor markers in breast and colorectal cancer. J Clin Oncol 1996; 14: 2843-77
2   Gasparini G (guest editor). Prognostic variables in node-negative and node-positive breast cancer – Part I & II. Breast Cancer Res Treat 1998; 51, 52 (special issues)
3   Clark GM. Do we really need prognostic factors for breast cancer? Breast Cancer Res Treat 1994; 30: 117-26

4   Amadori D, Silvestrini R. Prognostic and predictive value of thymidine labelling index in breast cancer. Breast Cancer Res Treat 1998; 51: 267-81

5   Gardin G, Alama A, Rosso R et al. Relationship of variations in tumor cell kinetics induced by primary chemotherapy to tumor regression and prognosis in locally advanced breast cancer. Breast Cancer Res Treat 1994; 32: 311-8

6   Hietänen P, Blomqvist C, Wasenius VM, et al. Do DNA ploidy and S-phase fraction in primary tumor predict the response to chemotherapy in metastatic breast cancer? Br J Cancer 1995; 71: 1029-32

7   Stål O, Nordenskjold B. S-phase fraction and survival benefit from adjuvant chemotherapy and radiotherapy of breast cancer. Br J Cancer 1994; 70: 1258-63

8   Stål O, Sullivan S, Wringen S et al. c-erbB-2 expression and benefit from adjuvant chemotherapy and radiotherapy of breast cancer. Eur J Cancer 1995; 31A: 2185-90

9   Paik S, Bryant J, Park C et al. ErbB-2 and response to doxorubicin in patients with axillary lymph node-positive, hormone receptor-negative breast cancer. J Natl Cancer Inst 1998; 90: 1361-70

10   Thor AD, Berry DA, Budman DR et al. ErbB-2, p53, and efficacy of adjuvant therapy in lymph node-positive breast cancer. J Natl Cancer Inst 1998; 90: 1346-60

11   Aas T, Børresen AL, Geisler S et al. Specific P53 mutations are associated with de novo resistance to doxorubicin in breast cancer patients. Nature Med 1996; 2: 811-4

12   Elledge RM, Gray R, Mansour E et al. Accumulation of p53 protein as a possible predictor of response to adjuvant combination chemotherapy with cyclophosphamide, methotrexate, fluorouracil, and prednisone for breast cancer. J Natl Cancer Inst 1995; 87: 1254-6

13   Krajewski S, Blomqvist C, Franssila K et al. Reduced expression of proapoptotic gene bax is associated with poor response rates to combination chemotherapy and shorter survival in women with metastatic breast adenocarcinoma. Cancer Res 1995; 55: 4471-8

14   Dowsett M. Improved prognosis for biomarkers in breast cancer. The Lancet 1998; 351: 1753-4

15   Bottini A, Berruti A, Bersiga A et al. Effect of neoadjuvant chemotherapy on Ki67 labelling index, c-erbB-2 expression and steroid hormone receptor status in human breast tumours. Anticancer Res 1996; 16: 3105-10

16   Daidone MG, Silvestrini R, Luisi A et al. Changes in biological markers after primary chemotherapy for breast cancers. Int J Cancer 1995; 61: 301-5

17   Ellis PA, Smith IE, McCarthy K, Detre S, Salter J, Dowsett M. Preoperative chemotherapy induces apoptosis in early breast cancer. The Lancet 1997; 349: 849

18   Baldini E, Giannessi PG, Collecchi P et al. Effects of primary chemotherapy on proliferative activity, IGF-1R and bcl2 expression in locally advanced breast cancer (Meeting abstract). Proc ASCO 1996; 15: A139

19   Briffod M, Tubiana-Hulin M, Spyratos F et al. Fine-needle cytopunctures for early prediction of tumor response to preoperative chemotherapy in 94 operable breast carcinomas (Meeting abstract). Proc ASCO 1995; 14: A261

20   Chevillard S, Pouillart P, Beldjord C et al. Sequential assessment of multidrug resistance phenotype and measurement of S-phase fraction as predictive markers of breast cancer response to neoadjuvant chemotherapy. Cancer 1996; 77: 292-300

21   Cocconi G, Guazzi A, Nizzoli R et al. Fine needle aspiration (FNA) cytology assessment of biological parameters and relationship with response to primary chemotherapy (CR) in operable breast carcinoma (BC). A biological study parallel to a randomized clinical trial (Meeting abstract). Proc ASCO 1996; 15: A46

22   Collecchi P, Baldini E, Giannessi P et al. Primary chemotherapy in locally advanced breast cancer (LABC): effects on tumour proliferative activity, bcl-2 expression and the relationship between tumour regression and biological markers. Eur J Cancer 1998; 34: 1701-4

23 Ellis PA, Smith IE, Detre S et al. Reduced apoptosis and proliferation and increased Bcl-2 in residual breast cancer following preoperative chemotherapy. Breast Cancer Res Treat 1998; 48: 107-16

24 Frassoldati A, Adami F, Banzi C, Criscuolo M, Piccinini L, Silingardi V. Changes of biological features in breast cancer cells determined by primary chemotherapy. Breast Cancer Res Treat 1997; 44: 185-92

25 Honkoop AH, Pinedo HM, De Jong JS et al. Effects of chemotherapy on pathologic and biologic characteristics of locally advanced breast cancer. Am J Clin Pathol 1997; 107: 211-8

26 Honkoop AH, van Diest PJ, de Jong JS et al. Prognostic role of clinical, pathological and biological characteristics in patients with locally advanced breast cancer. Br J Cancer 1998; 77: 621-6

27 Moll UM, Chumas J. Morphologic effects of neoadjuvant chemotherapy in locally advanced breast cancer. Pathol Res Practice 1997; 193: 187-96

28 Pierga JY, Lainé-Bidron C, Beuzeboc P, De Crémoux P, Pouillart P, Magdelénat H. Plasminogen activator inhibitor-1 (PAI-1) is not related to response to neoadjuvant chemotherapy in breast cancer. Br J Cancer 1997; 76: 537-40

29 Akashi-Tanaka S, Tsuda H, Fukuda H, Watanabe T, Fukutomi T. Prognostic value of histopathological therapeutic effects and mitotic index in locally advanced breast cancers after neoadjuvant chemotherapy. Jpn J Clin Oncol 1996; 26: 201-6

30 Bonetti A, Zaninelli M, Rodella S et al. Tumor proliferative activity and response to first-line chemotherapy in advanced breast carcinoma. Breast Cancer Res Treat 1996; 38: 289-97

31 Bonetti A, Zaninelli M, Leone R et al. Bcl-2 but not p53 expression is associated with resistance to chemotherapy in advanced breast cancer. Clin Cancer Res 1998; 4: 2331-6

32 Bottini A, Berruti A, Bersiga A et al. Cytotoxic and antiproliferative activity of the CMF regimen administered in association with tamoxifen as primary chemotherapy in breast cancer patients. Int J Oncol 1998; 13: 385-90

33 MacGrogan G, Mauriac L, Durand M et al. Primary chemotherapy in breast invasive carcinoma: predictive value of the immunohistochemical detection of hormonal receptors, p53, c-erbB-2, Mib1, pS2 and GSTπ. Br J Cancer 1996; 74: 1458-65

34 Makris A, Powles TJ, Dowsett M, Allred C. P53 protein overexpression and chemosensitivity in breast cancer. Lancet 1995; 345: 1181-2

35 Mathieu MC, Koscielny S, Le Bihan ML, Spielmann M, Arriagada R. p53 protein expression and chemosensitivity in breast cancer. Lancet 1995; 345: 1182

36 Paulsen T, Aas T, Børresen AL, Varhaug JE, Lønning PE, Akslen LA. Angiogenesis does not predict clinical response to doxorubicin monotherapy in patients with locally advanced breast cancer. Int J Cancer (Pred Oncol) 1997; 74: 138-40

37 Remvikos Y, Mosseri V, Asselain B et al. S-phase fractions of breast cancer predict overall and post-relapse survival. Eur J Cancer 1997; 33: 581-6

38 Rozan S, Vincent-Salomon A, Zafrani B et al. No significant predictive value of c-erbB-2 or p53 expression regarding sensitivity to primary chemotherapy or radiotherapy in breast cancer. Int J Cancer (Pred Oncol) 1998; 79: 27-33

39 Wang CS, LaRue H, Fortin A, Gariepy G, Tetu B. Mdr 1 mRNA expression by RT-PCR in patients with primary breast cancer submitted to neoadjuvant therapy. Breast Cancer Res Treat 1997; 45: 63-74

40 Willsher PC, Pinder SE, Gee JMW et al. c-erbB2 expression predicts response to preoperative chemotherapy for locally advanced breast cancer. Anticancer Res 1998; 18: 3695-8

41 Fernando IN, Titley JC, Powles TJ et al. Measurement of S-phase fraction and ploidy in sequential fine-needle aspirates from primary human breast tumors treated with tamoxifen. Br J Cancer 1994; 70: 1211-6

42 Jacob TW, Siziopikou KP, Prioleau JE, Raza S, Baum JK, Hayes DF, Schnitt SJ. Do prognostic marker studies on core needle biopsy specimens of breast carcinoma accurately reflect the marker status of the tumor? Modern Pathol 1998; 11: 259-64

43 Bonadonna G, Veronesi U, Brambilla C et al. Primary chemotherapy to avoid mastectomy in tumors with diameters of three centimeters or more. J Natl Cancer Inst 1990; 82: 1539-45

44 Silvestrini R (on behalf of the SICCAB Group for Quality Control of Cell Kinetic Determination). Feasibility and reproducibility of the ^{3}H-thymidine labeling index in breast cancer. Cell Prolif 1991; 24: 437-45

45 Silvestrini R, Daidone MG, Del Bino G et al. Prognostic significance of proliferative activity and ploidy in node-negative breast cancers. Ann Oncol 1993; 4: 213-9

46 Silvestrini R, Daidone MG, Luisi A et al. Biologic and clinicopathologic factors as indicators of specific relapse types in node-negative breast cancer. J Clin Oncol 1995; 13: 697-704

47 Silvestrini R, Benini E, Daidone MG et al. p53 as an independent prognostic marker in lymph node-negative breast cancer patients. J Natl Cancer Inst 1993; 85: 965-70

48 Silvestrini R, Veneroni S, Daidone MG et al. The bcl-2 protein: a prognostic indicator strongly related to p53 protein in lymph node-negative breast cancer patients. J Natl Cancer Inst 1994; 86: 499-504

49 Costa A, Licitra L, Veneroni S et al. Biological markers as indicators of pathological response to primary chemotherapy in oral cavity cancers. Int J Cancer (Pred Oncol) 1998; 79: 619-23

50 Remvikos Y, Jouve M, Beuzeboc P, Viehl P, Magdelénat H, Pouillart P. Cell cycle modifications of breast cancers during neoadjuvant chemotherapy: a flow cytometry study on fine needle aspirates. Eur J Cancer 1993; 29A: 1843-8

51 Strasser A, Huang DCS, Vaux DL. The role of the bcl-2/ced-9 family in cancer and general implications of defects in cell death control for tumorigenesis and resistance to chemotherapy. Biochim Biophys Acta 1997; 1333: F151-78

52 Ribeiro U, Finkelstein SD, Safatle-Ribeiro AV et al. p53 sequence analysis predicts treatment response and outcome of patients with esophageal carcinoma. Cancer 1998; 83: 7-18

53 Bonadonna G, Valagussa P, Brambilla C et al. Primary chemotherapy in operable breast cancer: eight-year experience at the Milan Cancer Institute. J Clin Oncol 1998; 16: 93-100

54 Righetti SC, Della Torre G, Pilotti S et al. A comparative study of p53 gene mutations, protein accumulation and response to cisplatin-based chemotherapy in advanced ovarian carcinoma. Cancer Res 1996; 56: 689-93

55 Weller M. Predicting response to cancer chemotherapy: the role of p53. Cell Tissue Res 1998; 292: 435-45

56 Amadori D, Volpi A, Nanni O et al. Prospective use of tumor proliferative activity for adjuvant therapy in node-negative breast cancer patients. Cell Prolif 1997; 30: 467

57 O'Reilly SM, Camplejohn RS, Millis RR, Rubens RD, Richards MA. Proliferative activity, histological grade and benefit from adjuvant chemotherapy in node positive breast cancer. Eur J Cancer 1990; 26: 1035-8

58 Zambetti M, Bonadonna G, Valagussa P, Bignami P. Adjuvant cyclophosphamide, methotrexate and fluorouracil in node-negative and estrogen receptor-negative breast cancer. Updated results. Ann Oncol 1996; 7: 481-5

59 Oltvai Z, Milliman C, Korsmeyer SJ. Bcl-2 heterodimerizes in vivo with a conserved homolog, Bax, that accelerates programmed cell death. Cell 1993; 74: 609-19

60 Daidone MG, Luisi A, Veneroni S, Benini E, Silvestrini R. Clinical studies of bcl-2 and treatment benefit in breast cancer patients. Endocrine Related Cancer 1999 (in press)

ESO Scientific Updates, Vol. 4
Primary Medical Therapy for Breast Cancer
A. Howell and M. Dowsett, editors
© 1999 Elsevier Science B.V. All rights reserved

TP53 as a Predictor of Response to Chemotherapy in Breast Cancer

Per Eystein Lønning[1], Hilde Johnsen[2], Stephanie Geisler[1], Turid Aas[3], Birgitte Smith-Sørensen[2], Lars-Andreas Akslen[4] and Anne-Lise Børresen-Dale[2]

1   Department of Medicine, Section of Oncology, Haukeland University Hospital, Bergen
2   Department of Genetics, The Norwegian Radiumhospital, Oslo
3   Department of Surgery and
4   Department of Pathology, The Gade Institute, Haukeland University Hospital, Bergen, Norway

Introduction

Resistance to systemic therapy (endocrine manipulation and chemotherapy) is the main obstacle to successful cancer treatment and the cause of death of the large majority of cancer patients. Despite the use of endocrine therapy for a century and the use of modern chemotherapy for three decades, only during recent years have we moved towards an understanding of the possible mechanisms of chemoresistance. We owe this to the rapidly developing knowledge in the field of molecular biology, which has provided new insight into the mechanisms controlling cell growth and, in particular, the mechanisms of programmed cell death, apoptosis.

This chapter reviews the influence of TP53 function on the efficacy of chemotherapy and discusses our own results and ongoing research programme evaluating the predictive value of mutations of TP53 and other genes for chemoresistance in breast cancer.

p53 as an executor of growth arrest and/or cell death in response to genotoxic damage

p53 (the protein encoded by the TP53 gene) plays a key role in inducing cellular responses to genotoxic damage. It activates downstream proteins (Fig. 1) involved in cell cycle arrest (p21), modulates genes involved in apoptosis (e.g.

Address for correspondence: P.E. Lønning, Department of Medicine, Section of Oncology, Haukeland University Hospital, 5021 Bergen, Norway. Tel: +47-55-972010, fax: +47-55-972046, e-mail: plon@haukeland.no

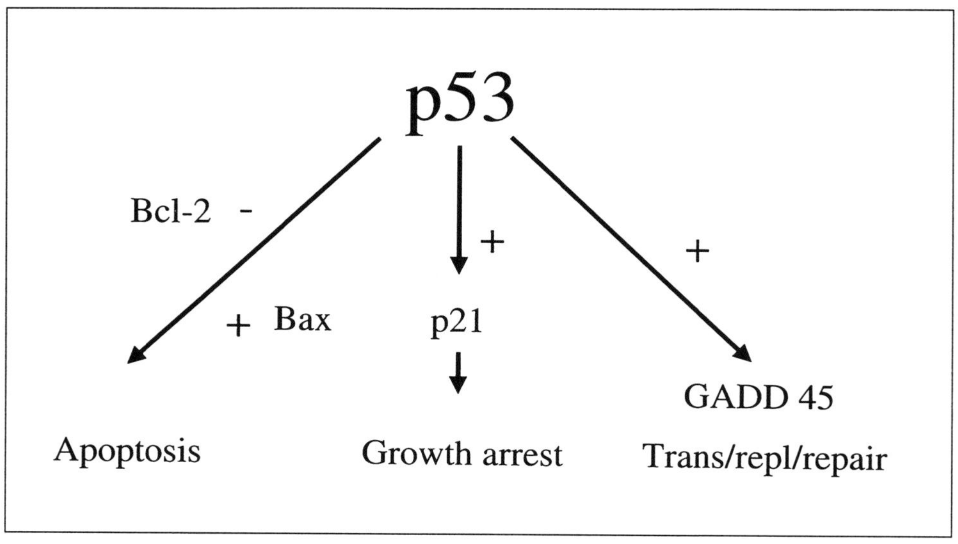

Fig. 1. Downstream genes activated by TP53.

bax) or DNA repair enzymes (e.g. GADD 45, reviewed in [1]). In addition, it may modulate the expression of several other genes including Fas [2], the type-I IGF-receptor and the IGF-binding protein IGFBP-3 [3,4]. Finally, p53 has been shown to exert functions that are independent of transcription, such as enhancing trafficking of Fas to the cell membrane [5].

The main pathways and downstream genes involved in p53-mediated growth arrest have been known for some time (Fig. 2), although new information has recently emerged [6-8], for example the role of the p14^{ARF} protein (the human homologue of murine p19^{ARF}) and the finding that p16, in addition to influencing the functional status of the retinoblastoma protein (pRB) by inhibiting the cyclin D complex, also downregulates pRB expression. By contrast, the interplay between p53 and other genes with respect to apoptosis is poorly understood. Several mechanisms, such as downregulation of the anti-apoptotic gene bcl-2 [9], upregulation of the pro-apoptotic gene bax [10], induction of the KILLER/DR5 receptor or Fas [11,12] as well as modulation of the IGF-system [3,4,13,14] have been proposed, but the potential contribution of the different mechanisms to the execution of apoptosis is currently unclear. Many of the findings reported are contradictory, and it is likely that cell type, as well as the experimental conditions *in vitro*, may have influenced the results.

Similarly, the mechanism(s) deciding whether p53 should cause growth arrest or induce apoptosis is poorly understood, and it is not clear at all whether these mechanisms are mutually exclusive, with growth arrest preventing apoptosis, or are activated in concert, or whether growth arrest actually may be a prerequisite for apoptosis [15-18]. Thus, p53-activated apoptosis with [19] or

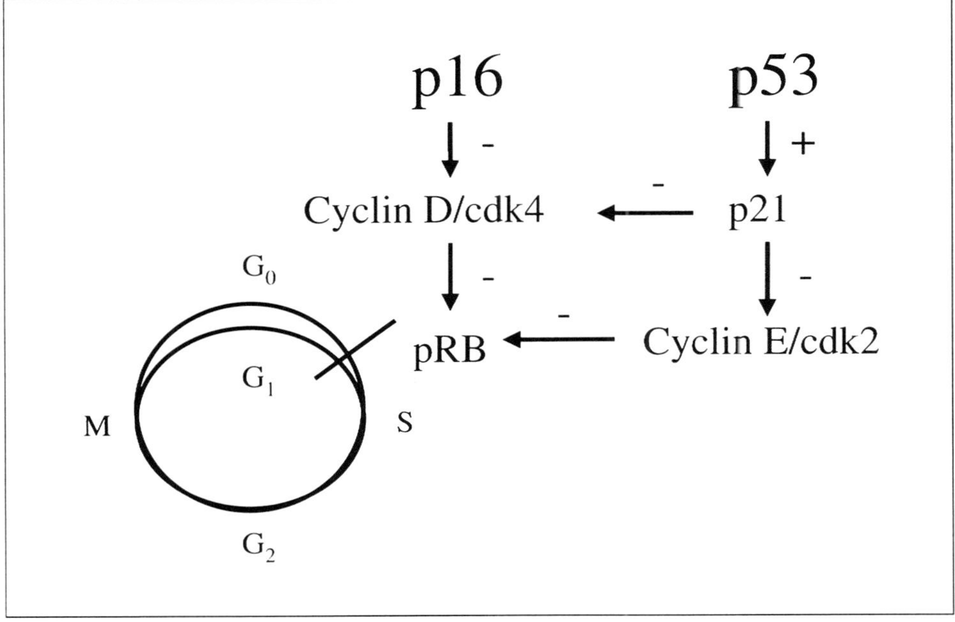

Fig. 2. TP53-dependent induction of cell cycle arrest.

without [20] concomitant activation of the p21 gene has been described by some authors, while others have shown expression of p21 to inhibit apoptosis [21]. Likewise, conflicting evidence has linked Fas to p53 for induction of apoptosis [5,22-26].

Notably, activation of the TP53 gene is not mandatory for apoptosis: recent studies have demonstrated apoptosis in p53-deficient cell lines obtained from different tissues in response to radiation as well as cytotoxic drugs [27-32]. This may be related to the type of toxic agent; there is evidence that apoptosis in response to treatment with taxanes is mediated through the TNF-alpha receptor and is enhanced by loss of p53 function [31,33].

TP53 activation

While the downstream pathways from p53, at least with respect to cell cycle arrest, are partly understood, an understanding of the mechanisms responsible for activating p53 in response to genotoxic stress has only recently been obtained. The p53 protein binds to its DNA consensus element as a tetramer [34]. Certain amino acids as well as some structural domains (the L2 and L3 loops, chelating a zinc ion) have been found to be critical to DNA binding, while other amino acids play a key role in stabilising the tertiary structure of the p53 protein [35].

In addition, p53 binds to other proteins like the mdm2 and the CBP/p300 complex. Expression of the mdm2 gene is known to be regulated by p53 in a feedback loop. While p53 has been shown to induce expression of the mdm2 gene [36], the mdm2 protein represses the function of p53 [37], conceals the p53 activation domain [38] and accelerates p53 degradation [39]. The finding that mutated p53 protein accumulates in the cell has been attributed to defective degradation, possibly due to defective induction of the mdm2 gene and lack of protein binding.

Phosphorylation appears to be a critical step in p53 activation in response to physical stress [40]. Several amino acid residues in the p53 protein undergo phosphorylation by different phosphokinases [41]. Recently, the protein encoded by the ataxia telangiectasia gene (ATM) was found to phosphorylate the p53 protein at Ser15 in response to radiation, but also following treatment with an antibiotic intercalating DNA [42,43]. Other types of genotoxic stress, like UV radiation, seem to activate p53 phosphorylation by activating other kinases [44]. Phosphorylation of p53 at Ser15 further activates acetylation of its carboxy terminal, which has been shown to activate sequence-specific DNA binding [45], and enhances p53 binding to the CBP/p300 protein complex [46]; this may be an important mechanism for transcriptional activation. While the mechanisms activating TP53 in response to cytotoxic therapy have not been fully elucidated, evidence suggests that phosphorylation of the p53 protein may be of importance. Thus, p53 has been reported to be phosphorylated at Ser4, 6 and 9 by casein kinase I in response to treatment with etoposide, and at the Ser15 site in response to treatment with the DNA-intercalating antibiotic neocarzinostatin [42]. Considering the emerging knowledge about the role of p53 in inducing cell death in response to anticancer therapy, it is reasonable to postulate that defects in TP53-activating mechanisms, in addition to mutations of the gene, also may contribute to therapy resistance in malignant diseases.

Mutations in the TP53 gene in human cancers

TP53 is the most frequently mutated gene in human cancers [47]. While an inherited alteration in the TP53 gene was the first genetic alteration accounting for a familial cancer syndrome, the Li-Fraumeni syndrome [48], germline mutation of the TP53 gene is a rare event among breast cancer patients without a family history of the Li-Fraumeni syndrome [49].

Initially thought to be an oncogene [50], p53 detected by immunostaining later proved to be mutated variants of a protein acting as a tumour suppressor [51]. Detection of TP53 mutations may be performed at the genomic level (CDGE, SSCP or sequencing); alternatively, many studies have used p53 immunostaining as a surrogate marker for TP53 mutations. While there is a significant correlation between TP53 mutations and p53 immunoreaction, a considerable number of tumours harbouring TP53 mutations do not stain for p53 expression [52,53]. In some cases nonsense mutations may imply loss of protein expression or deletion of part of the protein, including the epitopes the antibody is directed to. Also, it is known that many p53 point mutations may cause alterations in p53 tertiary structure expressing different epitopes compared to the normal protein, and antibodies specifically staining normal or mutated p53 protein have been developed [54,55]. However, the staining pattern may be unpredictable; for example, we have shown that the antibody D07 directed at an epitope in the N-terminal domain did not stain p53 proteins harbouring point mutations in locations like codon 190 and 249 [52]. Likewise, there is evidence that conformational status and immunostaining may vary due to intracellular location of the p53 protein, with differences between nuclear and cytoplasmic locations [56]. While TP53 mutations may be detected in formalin-fixed, paraffin-embedded tissue, the quality of such analysis does not reach the same standard as investigations conducted on snap-frozen tissue. Conversely, p53 immunostaining works well on paraffin-embedded archival material, which explains the popularity and widespread use of this method. The price of this "convenience", however, could be erroneous results and conclusions (see below).

Finally, there is emerging evidence that different types of TP53 mutations may have different biological functions. While mutations (in combination with loss of the normal allele) would be expected to cause loss of p53 function, some mutants still express specific DNA binding to a variable degree [55] and DNA binding may be enhanced by antibodies binding to the N-terminal domain of the p53 protein [57]. Furthermore, mutants have been shown to express a dominant negative function by driving the normal p53 protein into a mutant conformation [58] or to express gain of function, either by binding to alternative DNA sites [59] or through effects that seem to be independent of DNA binding [60,61].

p53 as a prognostic factor in breast cancer

Numerous studies have evaluated p53 status as a prognostic factor in breast cancer [62-66]. Interestingly, these studies revealed not only mutations in the TP53 gene but also expression of the p53 protein to predict a poor prognosis in node-negative as well as node-positive breast cancer patients. As most node-negative patients in these series were not exposed to adjuvant systemic therapy (specifically stated in [66]), such findings support the concept that p53 alterations have a prognostic impact independent of therapy.

Notably, while most studies report a prognostic impact of p53 alterations in breast cancer, whether determined by immunostaining or genomic analysis, determination of TP53 mutations seems to be superior to immunostaining in this respect [53,67], an observation recently made in relation to head and neck cancers as well [68]. Furthermore, mutations located in domains critical to DNA binding seem to predict a particularly poor prognosis in breast cancer patients [69,70].

TP53 mutations as a cause of chemoresistance in breast cancer

The importance of TP53 alterations for chemoresistance in breast cancer is controversial. Apart from some exceptions [71,72], most studies have failed to confirm a statistically significant relationship between immunostaining for the p53 protein and breast cancer resistance to chemotherapy in the adjuvant as well as neoadjuvant or advanced settings [73-80]. At first glance, the fact that similar observations have been made in a substantial number of studies evaluating different chemotherapy regimens administered in different clinical settings may seem convincing, refuting a key role of p53 status in the effectiveness of chemotherapy in this disease. However, our data question the validity of using immunohistochemistry as a surrogate marker for TP53 mutations when evaluating the predictive value of TP53 alterations for chemoresistance, as a number of tumours harbouring TP53 mutations associated with chemoresistance did not show immunostaining for p53 [52].

Studies evaluating the predictive value of p53 status for chemosensitivity with the use of immunostaining in other solid tumours obtained variable results [81-86]. By contrast, several studies evaluating TP53 mutations at the gene level revealed a predictive impact on response to different cytotoxic regimens in most haematological malignancies [87-90].

In 1991 we implemented a protocol treating patients with locally advanced (T3/4 and/or N2) breast carcinomas without (stage III) or with limited distant metastasis (stage IV) with preoperative doxorubicin administered as a weekly monotherapy schedule of 14 mg/m^2. This regimen has been in common use in our department for treatment of metastatic breast cancer with an acceptable response rate and good tolerability, also among senior patients [91]. Expecting many patients with stage III disease to be old (median age 64 years), we considered it justified to implement this treatment in the presurgical setting for this patient group.

The principal scientific aim of our study was to explore biological factors predicting primary resistance to chemotherapy in breast cancer. Due to the fact that different chemotherapeutic agents commonly used for breast cancer, such as anthracyclines, 5-fluorouracil and cyclophosphamide, act by attacking different cellular processes, we found it reasonable to hypothesise that the mechanisms of resistance to these drugs could be different. Accordingly, we preferred a monotherapy regimen for this study. The protocol was approved by the ethical committee of our institute.

In 1996 a preliminary analysis of the data was performed. At this time 63 patients were available for clinical and biological evaluation. The results published so far [52,92,93] are presented below and in Table 1.

1) TP53 mutations were found to predict for primary resistance to doxorubicin monotherapy. This related to TP53 mutations in general (p <0.05), but became even more significant when specific mutations affecting the L2 or L3 domain were analysed separately (p <0.01).

Table 1. Response to and relapse following weekly adriamycin 14 mg/m^2 as primary therapy in breast cancer and TP53 status

	Stage III and IV (n = 63)			Stage III (n = 56)	
	PR/MC/SD	PD	p	Relapse or PD	
No TP53 mutation	43	2*		8/40	(20%)
TP53 mutation	14	4	<0.05[1]	11/16	(69%)
Mutation in L2/L3	7	4	<0.01[2]	8/10	(80%)

* one patient with PD had a p16 mutation

PR = partial response, MC = minimal change, SD = stable disease, PD = progressive disease.
p values obtained
1) by comparing TP53 mutations to no mutations and
2) by comparing mutations affecting the L2/L3 domains to no mutations and mutations affecting other parts of the p53 protein.

2) While p53 immunostaining correlated with TP53 mutation status and predicted for a shorter overall and disease-free survival (p = 0.01), it was not statistically correlated with primary resistance to chemotherapy.
3) Expression of p21 was correlated with p53 functional status but did not add any further information of predictive value.
4) A low histological grade and a low mitotic frequency both predicted for chemotherapy response (high malignancy grade and high mitotic index were associated with chemoresistance).

This protocol has recently been closed and we are now updating the results. A total of 92 patients are evaluable for primary response to chemotherapy. In addition to p53 status evaluated immunohistochemically and at the gene level, we are measuring allelic imbalance with respect to the TP53 gene as well as expression of HER-2, mutations and methylation status of the p16 gene, and expression of the cyclins and the retinoblastoma protein. Interestingly, one of the patients with progressive disease who did not have a TP53 mutation had a mutation of the p16 gene (Table 1); however, the possible contribution of this mutation to drug resistance is unclear.

The finding of a poor response in patients with a high histological grade may be surprising. However, in our updated analysis we now observe a significant correlation between high histological grade and TP53 mutations (p <0.001). Noteworthily, a poor response in metastatic breast cancer patients with a high histological grade has also been reported by other authors [79].

Some other studies have recently revealed a correlation between TP53 mutations and response to chemotherapy in breast cancer patients. Kandioler-Eckerberger and colleagues [94] showed TP53 mutations to be predictive of resistance to combined treatment with 5-fluorouracil, epirubicin and cyclophosphamide; interestingly, they also observed TP53 mutations to enhance sensitivity to the taxane paclitaxel, an observation in accordance with *in vitro* data [33]. Lizard-Nacol and colleagues [95] reported a significant correlation between p53 "alterations" defined as mutations or LOH and lack of response to a combination chemotherapy regimen, while Formenti and colleagues [96] reported a correlation between TP53 mutations and lack of response to combined treatment with 5-fluorouracil and radiotherapy.

Further investigations

While our results revealed specific mutations in the TP53 gene but also loss of heterozygosity to predict for primary resistance to a low-dose anthracycline monotherapy regimen, several questions remain to be addressed. Notably, some patients showing primary resistance to therapy did not reveal any mutations in their TP53 gene, and we are currently analysing these tumours for other possible genetic alterations that may explain their lack of response. Such alterations may be located up- or downstream in the TP53 pathways; alternatively, they may involve other genes that may induce apoptosis in a p53-independent manner, growth factor overexpression or local alterations in drug disposition.

Another intriguing question is what may be the rescue mechanism(s) in tumours harbouring TP53 mutations found to be over-represented among patients having progressive disease on therapy (e.g. mutations affecting the L2 and L3 domains). The fact that many of these patients and all patients with progressive disease in addition express an allelic imbalance in their tumour suggests neither a dominant negative nor a gain of function of these mutations to be the discriminative factor; rather, it may be consistent with the hypothesis that other defects in addition to the TP53 mutations may act in synergy to cause chemoresistance. While mutations affecting the L2/L3 domain were also seen to influence survival in our patients [53], it is not possible to deduce from our material whether this might be due to a survival advantage of cells harbouring specific mutations rendering them resistant to therapy or, alternatively, to a higher metastatic potential of TP53-mutated tumour cells *per se* [97] causing a larger micrometastatic burden, probably together with a more rapid regrowth of the mutated tumour cells [98].

Concepts for future studies

The state of the art of breast cancer therapy in 1999 may be defined as follows: Despite a continuous and important improvement of adjuvant therapy with respect to chemotherapy [99] as well as hormonal treatment [100], such therapies do not prevent relapse or death in the majority of patients receiving them. In metastatic breast cancer the therapeutic benefits are modest [101], and long-term survival is an exception [102]. While new drugs such as the taxanes [103] represent interesting new treatment modalities, there is no substantial evidence so far suggesting either new drugs or even aggressive chemotherapy with stem cell support [104,105] to change this scenario. In our opinion it is unlikely that the introduction of new drugs or their use in combination or sequential regimens may change this picture in the years to come.

The number of randomised trials evaluating different chemotherapy regimens is enormous; a Medline search using the key words "breast cancer" and "chemotherapy" gave more than 10,000 hits for the last 10 years. What do we expect to achieve from further randomised phase III trials of chemotherapy in breast cancer?

The conceptual background for conducting clinical trials on breast cancer therapy has changed substantially over the last decade. Following the appearance of the paper by Slamon and colleagues [106] numerous publications have revealed a prognostic impact of oncogenes and growth factors in breast cancer. While the predictive value of oestrogen and progesterone receptors for the response to endocrine therapy in breast cancer was established more than 20 years ago [107,108], we still lack predictive factors for the response to chemotherapy. The substantial new information emerging in the field of molecular biology provides the clinicians with the challenging question of whether "classical" randomised phase III studies randomising unselected patients are still feasible or are actually a waste of time and resources.

Chemoresistance is the main reason for therapeutic failure and death in cancer patients. Results from *in vitro* studies have suggested a substantial number of possible mechanisms of resistance; now it is up to the clinicians to test these hypotheses in the *in vivo* setting.

We argue that chemoresistance studies require a conceptual "rethinking" of the way we conduct our clinical trails. Such studies should be prospective and not be conducted retrospectively for a number of reasons:

1) **Patient groups.** To study predictive factors in the adjuvant setting in principle means to correlate outcome (relapse and/or death) with predictive factors in two treatment arms that show a different clinical benefit, to be able to distinguish the "predictive" from the "prognostic" effect. Such studies require a substantial number of patients. In addition, many patients receiving adjuvant therapy will receive chemotherapy as well as endocrine treatment. Thus, to evaluate chemoresistance, we believe studies on patients receiving primary chemotherapy or treatment for metastatic disease are more appropriate.

2) **Optimal tissue sampling.** Studies on molecular factors in relation to therapy response require optimal tissue sampling and handling. As paraffin-embedded tissue is inferior to nitrogen-frozen specimens for studying alterations at the DNA/RNA level, such studies require well-defined logistics for tissue collection and handling beyond routine collection of specimens.

3) **Treatment regimens.** We prefer to avoid combined treatment modalities such as the simultaneous use of endocrine treatment and chemotherapy. With regard to chemotherapy regimens it has long been established that polychemotherapy is superior to monodrug treatment. This was confirmed in a re-

cent overview analysis [101]; however, the difference between anthracycline monotherapy and combined treatment was marginal, if any. This concept is further supported by data from a recent randomised study [109]. Similarly, taxanes have been found effective and may be used as monotherapy in advanced breast cancer.

Given the findings in the literature about the lack of crossresistance between anthracyclines and taxanes, there must be different mechanisms of resistance to the two regimens. While combined regimens may improve the immediate response rate, this may be at the cost of overtreating a substantial number of patients for a long time (those resistant to one of the regimens); in addition, the requirement for dose reductions of each drug to limit toxicity may, in theory, deteriorate the response in some patients. To obtain more information on the critical issue of mechanisms of chemoresistance, we believe that studies exploring two such monotherapy regimens in sequence combined with tissue sampling are justified and may not deteriorate optimal therapy to the patient.

In addition to our laboratory investigations with respect to the study mentioned above, other protocols have been activated. In all these studies tumour tissue is collected and snap-frozen prior to therapy to test for possible mechanisms of resistance at the gene level. Thus, to test whether alterations in the TP53 gene predict resistance to low-dose anthracycline therapy only or may also be associated with a lack of response to anthracyclines administered at higher doses as well as to other drug regimens used in breast cancer, we are currently randomising patients with locally advanced breast cancer to epirubicin 90 mg/m^2 versus paclitaxel 200 mg/m^2, each regimen being administered at three-weekly intervals and with crossover to the alternative regimen in case of an unsatisfactory response. This study is currently running as a Norwegian national study. In addition, about 30 patients with locally advanced breast cancer have received treatment with 5-fluorouracil (1000 mg/m^2) and mitomycin (6 mg/m^2) every third week [110] following surgical biopsies with snap-frozen tissue. Finally, we are conducting prospective studies in patients with metastatic breast cancer treated with epirubicin or docetaxel. It is our hope that the results of these studies may improve our understanding of the mechanisms of chemoresistance in breast cancer.

Acknowledgement

Our work was funded by the Norwegian Cancer Society.

References

1   Bergh J. Determination and use of p53 in the management of cancer patients, with special focus on breast cancer - A review. In: Klijn JGM, ed. Prognostic and predictive value of p53. ESO Scientific Updates, Vol 1. Amsterdam: Elsevier Science B.V. 1997; 35-50

2   Miller M, Wilder S, Bannasch D et al. p53 activates the CD95 (APO-1/Fas) gene in response to DNA damage by anticancer drugs. J Exp Med 1998; 188: 2033-45

3   Werner H, Karnieli E, Rauscher FJ, Leroith D. Wild-type and mutant p53 differentially regulate transcription of the insulin-like growth factor I receptor gene. Proc Natl Acad Sci USA 1996; 93: 8318-23

4   Buckbinder L, Talbott R, Velasco-Miguel S et al. Induction of the growth inhibitor IGF-binding protein 3 by p53. Nature 1995; 377: 646-9

5   Bennett M, Macdonald K, Chan SW, Luzio JP, Simari R, Weissberg P. Cell surface trafficking of Fas: A rapid mechanism of p53-mediated apoptosis. Science 1998; 282: 290-3

6   Pomerantz J, SchreiberAgus N, Liegeois NJ et al. The Ink4a tumor suppressor gene product, p19(Arf), interacts with MDM2 and neutralizes MDM2's inhibition of p53. Cell 1998; 92: 713-23

7   Bates S, Phillips AC, Clark PA et al. p14(ARF) links the tumour suppressors RB and p53. Nature 1998; 395: 124-5

8   Fang X, Jin X, Xu H et al. Expression of p16 induces transcriptional downregulation of the RB gene. Oncogene 1998; 16: 1-8

9   Haldar S, Negrini M, Monne M, Sabbioni S, Croce CM. Down-regulation of bcl-2 by p53 in breast cancer cells. Cancer Res 1994; 54: 2095-7

10   Mitry RR, Sarraf CE, Wu CG, Pignatelli M, Habib NA. Wild-type p53 induces apoptosis in Hep3B through up-regulation of bax expression. Lab Invest 1997; 77: 369-78

11   Wu GS, Burns TF, McDonald III ER et al. Killer/DR5 is a DNA damage-inducible p53-regulated death receptor gene. Nature Genetics 1997; 17: 141-3

12   Sheard MA, Vojtesek B, Janakova L, Kovarik J, Zaloudik J. Up-regulation of fas (CD95) in human p53(wild-type) cancer cells treated with ionizing radiation. Int J Cancer 1997; 73: 757-62

13   Baserga R, Resnicoff M, Dambrosio C, Valentinis B. The role of the IGF-I receptor in apoptosis. Vitamins and Hormones Advances in Research and Applications 1997; 53: 65-98

14   Rajah R, Valentinis B, Cohen P. Insulin like growth factor (IGF)-binding protein-3 induces apoptosis and mediates the effects of transforming growth factor-beta 1 on programmed cell death through a p53- and IGF-independent mechanism. J Biol Chem 1997; 272: 12181-8

15   Erhardt JA, Pittman RN. p21(WAF1) induces permanent growth arrest and enhances differentiation, but does not alter apoptosis in PC12 cells. Oncogene 1998; 16: 443-51

16   Gansauge S, Nussler AK, Beger HG, Gansauge F. Nitric oxide-induced apoptosis in human pancreatic carcinoma cell lines is associated with a G(1)-arrest and an increase of the cyclin-dependent kinase inhibitor p21(WAF1/CIP1). Cell Growth Differ 1998; 9: 611-7

17   Oh WJ, Kim WH, Kang KH, Kim TY, Kim MY, Choi KH. Induction of p21 during ceramide-mediated apoptosis in human hepatocarcinoma cells. Cancer Lett 1998; 129: 215-22

18   Suzuki A, Tsutomi Y, Akahane K, Araki T, Miura M. Resistance to Fas-mediated apoptosis: activation of caspase 3 is regulated by cell cycle regulator p21(WAF1) and IAP gene family ILP. Oncogene 1998; 17: 931-9

19   Gansauge S, Gansauge F, Gause H, Poch B, Schoenberg MH, Beger HG. The induction of apoptosis in proliferating human fibroblasts by oxygen radicals is associated with a p53- and p21(WAF1CIP1) induction. FEBS Lett 1997; 404: 6-10

84   P.E. Lønning, H. Johnsen, S. Geisler et al.

20   Attardi LD, Lowe SW, Brugarolas J, Jacks T. Transcriptional activation by p53, but not induction of the p21 gene, is essential for oncogene-mediated apoptosis. Embo J 1996; 15: 3693-701
21   Gorospe M, Cirielli C, Wang XT, Seth P, Capogrossi MC, Holbrook NJ. p21 (Waf1/Cip1) protects against p53-mediated apoptosis of human melanoma cells. Oncogene 1997; 14: 929-35
22   Tolomeo M, Dusonchet L, Meli M et al. The CD95/CD95 ligand system is not the major effector in anticancer drug-mediated apoptosis. Cell Death Differentiation 1998; 5: 735-42
23   Muller M, Strand S, Hug H et al. Drug-induced apoptosis in hepatoma cells is mediated by the CD95 (APO-1/Fas) receptor/ligand system and involves activation of wild-type p53. J Clin Invest 1997; 99: 403-13
24   Fuchs EJ, McKenna KA, Bedi A. p53-dependent DNA damage-induced apoptosis requires Fas/APO-1-independent activation of CPP32 beta. Cancer Res 1997; 57: 2550-4
25   Reinke V, Lozano G. The p53 targets mdm2 and Fas are not required as mediators of apoptosis in vivo. Oncogene 1997; 15: 1527-34
26   Miyake H, Hara I, Gohji K, Arakawa S, Kamidono S. p53 modulation of Fas/Apo-1 mediated apoptosis in a human renal cell carcinoma cell line. Int J Oncol 1998; 12: 469-73
27   Ahmed MM, Sells SF, Venkatasubbarao K et al. Ionizing radiation-inducible apoptosis in the absence of p53 linked to transcription factor EGR-1. J Biol Chem 1997; 272: 33056-61
28   Yu YJ, Little JB. p53 is involved in but not required for ionizing radiation-induced caspase-3 activation and apoptosis in human lymphoblast cell lines. Cancer Res 1998; 58: 4277-81
29   Clarke AR, Purdie CA, Harrison DJ et al. Thymocyte apoptosis induced by p53-dependent and independent pathways. Nature 1993; 362: 849-52
30   Jones JM, Attardi L, Godley LA et al. Absence of p53 in a mouse mammary tumor model promotes tumor cell proliferation without affecting apoptosis. Cell Growth Differ 1997; 8: 829-38
31   Lanni JS, Lowe SW, Licitra EJ, Liu JO, Jacks T. p53-independent apoptosis induced by paclitaxel through an indirect mechanism. Proc Natl Acad Sci USA 1997; 94: 9679-83
32   Strasser A, Harris AW, Jacks T, Cory S. DNA damage can induce apoptosis in proliferating lymphoid cells via p53-independent mechanisms inhibitable by Bcl-2. Cell 1994; 79: 329-39
33   Wahl AF, Donaldson KL, Fairchild C et al. Loss of normal p53 function confers sensitization to taxol by increasing G2/M arrest and apoptosis. Nature Med 1996; 2: 72-9
34   Cho Y, Gorina S, Jeffrey PD, Pavletich NP. Crystal structure of a p53 tumor suppressor-DNA complex: Understanding tumorigenic mutations. Science 1994; 265: 346-55
35   Wieczorek AM, Waterman JLF, Waterman MJF, Halazonetis TD. Structure-based rescue of common tumor-derived p53 mutants. Nature Med 1996; 2: 1143-6
36   Wu X, Bayle JH, Olson D, Levine AJ. The p53-mdm-2 autoregulatory feedback loop. Genes Devel 1993; 17: 1126-32
37   Thut CJ, Goodrich JA, Tjian R. Repression of p53-mediated transcription by MDM2: a dual mechanism. Gene Develop 1997; 11: 1974-86
38   Oliner JD, Pietenpol JA, Thiagalingam S, Gyuris J, Kinzler KW, Vogelstein B. Oncoprotein MDM2 conceals the activation domain of tumour suppressor p53. Nature 1993; 362: 857-60
39   Haupt Y, Maya R, Kazaz A, Oren M. Mdm2 promotes the rapid degradation of p53. Nature 1997; 387: 296-9
40   Steegenga WT, Vandereb AJ, Jochemsen AG. How phosphorylation regulates the activity of p53. J Mol Biol 1996; 263: 103-13

41 Meek DW, Campbell LE, Jardine LJ, Knippschild U, McKendrick L, Milne DM. Multi-site phosphorylation of p53 by protein kinases inducible by p53 and DNA damage. Biochem Soc Trans 1997; 25: 416-9

42 Banin S, Moyal L, Shieh SY et al. Enhanced phosphorylation of p53 by ATM in response to DNA damage. Science 1998; 281: 1674-7

43 Canman CE, Lim DS, Cimprich KA et al. Activation of the ATM kinase by ionizing radiation and phosphorylation of p53. Science 1998; 281: 1677-9

44 Kapoor M, Lozano G. Functional activation of p53 via phosphorylation following DNA damage by UV but not gamma radiation. Proc Natl Acad Sci USA 1998; 95: 2834-7

45 Gu W, Roeder RG. Activation of p53 sequence-specific DNA birding by acetylation of the p53 C-terminal domain. Cell 1997; 90: 595-606

46 Lambert PF, Kashanchi F, Radonovich MF, Shiekhattar R, Brady JN. Phosphorylation of p53 serine 15 increases interaction with CBP. J Biol Chem 1998; 273: 33048-53

47 Hollstein M, Rice K, Greenblatt MS et al. Database of p53 gene somatic mutations in human tumors and cell lines. Nucleic Acid Res 1994; 22: 3551-5

48 Garber JE, Goldstein AM, Kantor AF, Dreyfus MG, Fraumeni JF, Li FP. Follow-up study of twenty-four families with Li-Fraumeni syndrome. Cancer Res 1991; 51: 6094-7

49 Børresen A-L, Andersen TI, Garber J et al. Screening for germ line TP53 mutations in breast cancer patients. Cancer Res 1992; 52: 3234-6

50 Lane DP, Crawford LV. T antigen is bound to a host protein in SV 40-transformed cells. Nature 1979; 278: 261-3

51 Wang XW, Harris CC. TP53 tumour suppressor gene: Clues to molecular carcinogenesis and cancer therapy. Cancer Surv 1996; 28: 169-96

52 Aas T, Børresen A-L, Geisler S et al. Specific P53 mutations are associated with de novo resistance to doxorubicin in breast cancer patients. Nature Med 1996; 2: 811-4

53 Sjögren S, Inganäs M, Norberg T et al. The p53 gene in breast cancer: Prognostic value of complementary DNA sequencing versus immunohistochemistry. J Natl Cancer Inst 1996; 88: 173-82

54 Legros Y, Meyer A, Ory K, Soussi T. Mutations in p53 produce a common conformational effect that can be detected with a panel of monoclonal antibodies directed toward the central part of the p53 protein. Oncogene 1994; 9: 3689-94

55 Rolley N, Butcher S, Milner J. Specific DNA binding by different classes of human p53 mutants. Oncogene 1995; 11: 763-70

56 Danks MK, Whipple DO, McPake CR, Lu DY, Harris LC. Differences in epitope accessibility of p53 monoclonal antibodies suggest at least three conformations or states of protein binding of p53 protein in human tumor cell lines. Cell Death Differentiation 1998; 5: 678-86

57 Friedlander P, Legros Y, Soussi T, Prives C. Regulation of mutant p53 temperature-sensitive DNA binding. J Biol Chem 1996; 271: 25468-78

58 Chene P. In vitro analysis of the dominant negative effect of p53 mutants. J Mol Biol 1998; 281: 205-9

59 Müller BF, Paulsen D, Deppert W. Specific binding of MAR/SAR DNA-elements by mutant p53. Oncogene 1996; 12: 1941-52

60 Dittmer D, Pati S, Zambetti G et al. Gain of function mutations in p53. Nature Genet 1993; 4: 42-6

61 Gualberto A, Aldape K, Kozakiewicz K. An oncogenic form of p53 confers a dominant, gain-of-function phenotype that disrupts spindle checkpoint control. Proc Natl Acad Sci USA 1998; 95: 5166-71

62 Thor AD, Moore DHI, Edgerton SM et al. Accumulation of p53 tumor suppressor gene protein: An independent marker of prognosis in breast cancers. J Natl Cancer Inst 1992; 84: 845-55

86   P.E. Lønning, H. Johnsen, S. Geisler et al.

63   Thorlacius S, Börresen AL, Eyfjörd JE. Somatic p53 mutations in human breast carci-
      nomas in an Icelandic population: a prognostic factor. Cancer Res 1993; 53: 1637-41
64   Elledge RM, Fuqua SAW, Clark GM, Pujol P, Allred DC, McGuire WL. Prognostic sig-
      nificance of p53 gene alterations in node-negative breast cancer. Breast Cancer Res
      1993; 26: 225-35
65   Andersen TI, Holm R, Nesland JM, Heimdal KR, Ottestad L, Børresen AL. Prognostic
      significance of TP53 alterations in breast carcinoma. Br J Cancer 1993; 68: 540-8
66   Bergh J, Norberg T, Sjögren S, Lindgren A, Holmberg L. Complete sequencing of the p53
      gene provides prognostic information in breast cancer patients, particularly in rela-
      tion to adjuvant systemic therapy and radiotherapy. Nature Med 1995; 1: 1029-34
67   Thorlacius S, Thorgilsson B, Björnsson J et al. TP53 mutations and abnormal p53 pro-
      tein staining in breast carcinomas related to prognosis. Eur J Cancer 1995; 31A: 1856-
      61
68   Mineta H, Borg A, Dictor M, Wahlberg P, Akervall J, Wennerberg J. p53 mutation, but
      not p53 overexpression, correlates with survival in head and neck squamous cell car-
      cinoma. Br J Cancer 1998; 78: 1084-90
69   Børresen AL, Andersen TI, Eyfjörd JE et al. TP53 mutations and breast cancer progno-
      sis: Particularly poor survival rates for cases with mutations in the zinc-binding do-
      mains. Genes, Chromosomes & Cancer 1995; 14: 71-5
70   Berns EMJJ, van Staveren IL, Look MP, Smid M, Klijn JGM, Foekens JA. Mutations in
      residues of TP53 that directly contact DNA predict poor outcome in human primary
      breast cancer. Br J Cancer 1998; 77: 1130-6
71   Clahsen PC, van de Velde CJH, Duval C et al. p53 protein accumulation and response
      to adjuvant chemotherapy in premenopausal women with node-negative early breast
      cancer. J Clin Oncol 1998; 16: 470-9
72   Tetu B, Brisson J, Plante V, Bernard P. p53 and c-erbB-2 as markers of resistance to
      adjuvant chemotherapy in breast cancer. Modern Pathol 1998; 11: 823-30
73   Dublin EA, Miles DW, Rubens RD, Smith P, Barnes DM. p53 immunohistochemical
      staining and survival after adjuvant chemotherapy for breast cancer. Int J Cancer
      1997; 74: 605-8
74   Stål O, Askmalm MS, Wingren S et al. p53 expression and the result of adjuvant thera-
      py of breast cancer. Acta Oncol 1995; 34: 767-70
75   Elledge RM, Gray R, Mansour E et al. Accumulation of p53 protein as a possible pre-
      dictor of response to adjuvant combination chemotherapy with cyclophosphamide,
      methotrexate, fluorouracil, and prednisone for breast cancer. J Natl Cancer Inst 1995;
      87: 1254-6
76   Jacquemier J, Penault-Llorca F, Viens P et al. Breast cancer response to adjuvant che-
      motherapy in correlation with erbB2 and p53 expression. Anticancer Res 1994; 14:
      2773-8
77   MacGrogan G, Mauriac L, Durand M et al. Primary chemotherapy in breast invasive
      carcinoma: Predictive value of the immunohistochemical detection of hormonal recep-
      tors, p53, c-erbB-2, MiB1, pS2 and GST pi. Br J Cancer 1996; 74: 1458-65
78   Makris A, Powles TJ, Dowsett M et al. Prediction of response to neoadjuvant chemo-
      endocrine therapy in primary breast carcinomas. Clin Cancer Res 1997; 3: 593-600
79   Niskanen E, Blomqvist C, Franssila K, Hietanen P, Wasenius V-M. Predictive value of
      c-erbB-2, p53, cathepsin-D and histology of the primary tumour in metastatic breast
      cancer. Br J Cancer 1997; 76: 917-22
80   Thor AD, Berry DA, Budman DR et al. erbB-2, p53, and efficacy of adjuvant therapy
      in lymph node-positive breast cancer. J Natl Cancer Inst 1998; 90: 1346-60
81   Cascinu S, Graziano F, DelFerro E et al. Expression of p53 protein and resistance to
      preoperative chemotherapy in locally advanced gastric carcinoma. Cancer 1998; 83:
      1917-22

82   Rusch V, Klimstra D, Venkatraman E et al. Aberrant p53 expression predicts clinical resistance to cisplatin-based chemotherapy in locally advanced non-small cell lung cancer. Cancer Res 1995; 55: 5038-42

83   Kawasaki M, Nakanishi Y, Kuwano K, Takayama K, Kiyohara C, Hara N. Immuno-histochemically detected p53 and P-glycoprotein predict the response to chemotherapy in lung cancer. Eur J Cancer 1998; 34: 1352-7

84   Righetti SC, Torre GD, Pilotti S et al. A comparative study of p53 gene mutations, protein accumulation, and response to cisplatin-based chemotherapy in advanced ovarian carcinoma. Cancer Res 1996; 56: 689-93

85   Puglisi F, Di Loreto C, Panizzo R et al. Expression of p53 and bcl-2 and response to preoperative chemotherapy and radiotherapy for locally advanced squamous cell carcinoma of the oesophagus. J Clin Path 1996; 49: 456-9

86   Paradiso A, Rabinovich M, Vallejo C et al. p53 and PCNA expression in advanced colorectal cancer: Response to chemotherapy and long-term prognosis. Int J Cancer 1996; 69: 437-41

87   Diccianni MB, Yu J, Hsiao M, Mukherjee S, Shao L-E, Yu AL. Clinical significance of p53 mutations in relapsed T-cell acute lymphoblastic leukemia. Blood 1994; 84: 3105-2

88   Wattel E, Preudhomme C, Hecquet B et al. p53 mutations are associated with resistance to chemotherapy and short survival in hematologic malignancies. Blood 1994; 84: 3148-57

89   Preudhomme C, Dervite I, Wattel E et al. Clinical significance of p53 mutations in newly diagnosed Burkitt's lymphoma and acute lymphoblastic leukemia: A report of 48 cases. J Clin Oncol 1995; 13: 812-20

90   Ichikawa A, Kinoshita T, Watanabe T et al. Mutations of the p53 gene as a prognostic factor in aggressive B-cell lymphoma. N Engl J Med 1997; 337: 529-34

91   Gundersen S, Kvinnsland S, Klepp O, Kvaløy S, Lund E, Høst H. Weekly adriamycin versus VAC in advanced breast cancer. A randomized trial. Eur J Cancer Clin Oncol 1986; 22: 1431-4

92   Aas T, Geisler S, Paulsen T et al. Primary systemic treatment with weekly doxorubicin monotherapy in women with locally advanced breast cancer; clinical experience and parameters predicting outcome. Acta Oncol 1996; 35: 5-8

93   Ellis PA, Lønning PE, Børresen-Dale A-L et al. Absence of p21 expression is associated with abnormal p53 in human breast carcinomas. Br J Cancer 1997; 76: 480-5

94   Kandioler-Eckerberger D, Taucher S, Steiner B et al. p53 genotype and major response to anthracycline or paclitaxel based neoadjuvant treatment in breast cancer patients. Proc ASCO 1998; 17: 102a (Abstr. 392)

95   LizardNacol S, Coudert B, Riedinger JM, Fargeot P, Guerrin J. p53 gene alterations are associated with a decreased responsiveness to neoadjuvant chemotherapy in human breast cancer. Int J Oncol 1997; 10: 1203-7

96   Formenti SC, Dunnington G, Uzieli B et al. Original p53 status predicts for pathological response in locally advanced breast cancer patients treated preoperatively with continuous infusion 5-fluorouracil and radiation therapy. Int J Radiat Oncol Biol Phys 1997; 39: 1059-68

97   Navone NM, Labate ME, Troncoso P et al. p53 mutations in prostate cancer bone metastases suggest that selected p53 mutants in the primary site define foci with metastatic potential. J Urol 1999; 161: 304-8

98   Pegram MD, Finn RS, Arzoo K, Beryt M, Pietras RJ, Slamon DJ. The effect of HER-2/neu overexpression on chemotherapeutic drug sensitivity in human breast and ovarian cancer cells. Oncogene 1997; 15: 537-47

99   Group EBCTC. Polychemotherapy for early breast cancer: an overview of the randomised trials. Lancet 1998; 352: 930-42

100 Clarke M, Collins R, Davies C, Godwin J, Gray R, Peto R. Tamoxifen for early breast cancer: An overview of the randomised trials. Lancet 1998; 351: 1451-67

101 Fossati R, Confalonieri C, Torri V et al. Cytotoxic and hormonal treatment for metastatic breast cancer: A systematic review of published randomized trials involving 31,510 women. J Clin Oncol 1998; 16: 3439-60
102 Greenberg PAC, Hortobagyi GN, Smith TL, Ziegler LD, Frye DK, Buzdar AU. Long-term follow-up of patients with complete remission following combination chemotherapy for metastatic breast cancer. J Clin Oncol 1996; 14: 2197-205
103 Ravdin PM. Docetaxel (Taxotere) for the treatment of anthracycline-resistant breast cancer. Semin Oncol 1997; 24: 18-21
104 Garcia-Carbonero R, Hidalgo M, Paz-Arez L et al. Patient selection in high-dose chemotherapy trials: Relevance in high-risk breast cancer. J Clin Oncol 1997; 15: 3178-84
105 Rahman ZU, Frye DK, Buzdar AU et al. Impact of selection process on response rate and long-term survival of potential high-dose chemotherapy candidates treated with standard-dose doxorubicin-containing chemotherapy in patients with metastatic breast cancer. J Clin Oncol 1997; 15: 3171-7
106 Slamon DJ, Clark GM, Wong SG, Levin WJ, Ullrich A, McGuire WL. Human breast cancer: correlation of relapse and survival with amplification of the HER-2/neu oncogene. Science 1987; 235: 177-82
107 Jensen EV, DeSombre ER, Jungblut PP. Estrogen receptors in hormone-responsive tissues and tumors. In: Wissler RW, Dao TL, Wood S Jr, eds. Endogenous factors influencing host-tumor balance. University of Chicago Press 1967; 15-30
108 McGuire WL. Steroid receptors in human breast cancer. Cancer Res 1978; 38: 4289-91
109 Joensuu H, Holli K, Heikkinen M et al. Combination chemotherapy versus single-agent therapy as first- and second-line treatment in metastatic breast cancer: A prospective randomized trial. J Clin Oncol 1998; 16: 3720-30
110 Gundersen S, Kvinnsland S, Klepp O, Lund E, Hannisdal E, Høst H. Chemotherapy with or without high-dose medroxyprogesterone acetate in oestrogen-receptor-negative advanced breast cancer. Eur J Cancer 1992; 28: 390-4

ESO Scientific Updates, Vol. 4
Primary Medical Therapy for Breast Cancer
A. Howell and M. Dowsett, editors
© 1999 Elsevier Science B.V. All rights reserved

Neoadjuvant Endocrine Treatment: The Edinburgh Experience

William R. Miller, Thomas J. Anderson, R. Anthony Hawkins, Jeremy Keen and J. Michael Dixon

Edinburgh Breast Unit Research Group, Western General Hospital, Edinburgh, United Kingdom

Introduction

The Edinburgh Breast Unit has had a long experience of primary or "neoadjuvant" systemic treatment for breast cancer. In 1986 Forrest et al. [1] published a paper entitled "A human model for breast cancer". The title was chosen deliberately to emphasise that the strategy of switching the conventional sequence of "breast surgery followed by systemic therapy" produced a model system in which the tumour itself acted as a test-bed for drug-based regimes (in distinction to other forms of model systems in which drugs are tested *in vitro*). The approach was designed to produce potential clinical benefits by (i) downstaging large tumours so that ultimately more conservative surgery could be given and (ii) using knowledge of tumour sensitivity to a trial therapy to tailor rationally subsequent adjuvant treatment (even patients with non-responding tumours might benefit by avoiding the unnecessary side effects of an extended period of adjuvant treatment with an ineffective agent). However, the particular attraction of the approach extended beyond clinical benefits in that accessibility of the primary tumour meant that (i) its size could be precisely measured to provide accurate response data and (ii) sequential samples could be taken from the tumour before, during and after treatment. It was therefore possible to relate biological and molecular characteristics of the tumour to its clinical response as well as monitoring changes which occurred as a result of that response. The intent was to explore the endocrinology within the breast and its tumours and derive fundamental knowledge about the mechanisms of response/resistance to treatment, with the ultimate aims of identifying biological markers which predicted the response to treatment and eliciting changes which might be markers of acquired resistance.

Address for correspondence: W.R. Miller, Edinburgh Breast Unit Research Group, Western General Hospital, Edinburgh EH4 2XU, United Kingdom. Tel.: +44-131-5372505, fax +44-131-5372449, e-mail: wrmiller@srv0.med.ed.ac.uk

Table 1. Relationship between tumour oestrogen receptor status and response to primary endocrine therapy in 89 patients with breast cancer

	ER-poor	ER-rich
Responders	1	35
Non-responders	26	27

ER-poor is < 20 fmol/mg cytosol protein
ER-rich is > 20 fmol/mg cytosol protein

Response to endocrine therapy

In Edinburgh, two separate cohorts of patients were entered into studies of primary systemic therapy, viz. women with large primary tumours and elderly patients who wished to avoid surgery. Initially, patients were recruited for treatment irrespective of oestrogen receptor status (ER). However, as is shown in Table 1, only one of 27 ER-poor (<20 fmol/mg cytosol protein) tumours responded to various endocrine therapies (which included oophorectomy and LHRH agonists in premenopausal women and aminoglutethimide, 4-hydroxy-androstenedione and tamoxifen in postmenopausal patients). In contrast, 35 of 62 ER-rich tumours regressed within three months of treatment. Because of this, the decision was taken to restrict subsequent endocrine therapy to patients with oestrogen-receptor-rich tumours.

Rapidity of response to treatment was determined by serial ultrasound measurements in a series of 68 women older than 70 years with ER-rich tumours, all of whom were treated with tamoxifen. These results are summarised in Figure 1.

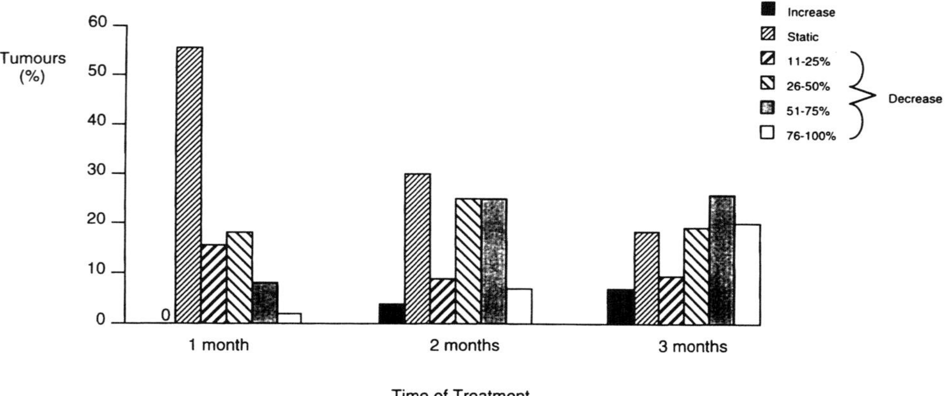

Fig. 1. Change in tumour volume as assessed by ultrasound at 1, 2 and 3 months in elderly patients treated with primary tamoxifen therapy.

Whilst the majority of tumours did not reduce in size in the first month, some did regress and occasional cancers showed a marked shrinkage. At two months the number of tumours remaining static was substantially reduced; several tumours increased in volume but most showed a substantial decrease in size (including all those which had responded at one month). This pattern was further accentuated at three months, a minority of tumours showing progression or stasis but most showing a volume reduction (again, all tumours responding at two months continued to do so at three months). The final incidence of response (>25% decrease in tumour volume) was 76%. Of these patients, 20 elected to continue tamoxifen treatment to six months. Amongst 16 initially responding tumours, 12 continued to decrease in size, three showed no further response but one tumour now showed evidence of progression. Of the four initially non-responders, one progressed, one remained static and two now showed evidence of response. It is clear that in this patient population, the majority of responses to tamoxifen occur within two to three months, but later responses can be seen. However, because of the emergence of progressive disease at six months, we decided to administer subsequent neoadjuvant endocrine therapy for a standard trial period of three months.

The level of oestrogen receptors in the tumours subdivided into responders and non-responders as assessed at one, two and three months, is shown in Figure 2. The range of ER concentrations was similar in groups of tumours either showing early response (at one month) or not. However, with increasing time of treatment, differences between responders and non-responders became apparent. At three months, the mean value for oestrogen receptors was significantly higher in the responding group; indeed, *all* tumours with levels greater than 200 fmol/mg cytosol protein showed a reduction in size with treatment, whereas tumours with values below this amount were equally likely to respond or not.

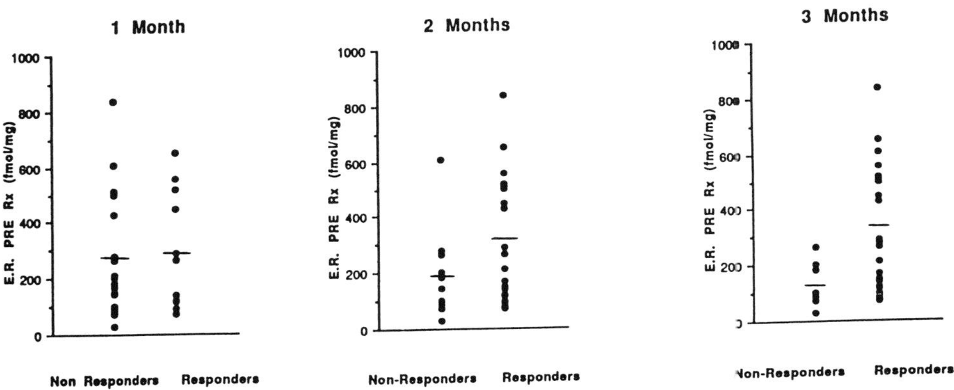

Fig. 2. Oestrogen receptor levels in breast cancers from elderly patients subdivided into response at 1, 2 and 3 months.

Despite this, there was a highly significant relationship between the degree of change in tumour size during treatment and the level of oestrogen receptors as measured by ELISA (Abbott ER-EIA) (Fig. 3a); interestingly the corresponding correlation with oestrogen receptor by immunohistochemistry on a fine needle aspirate (Abbott ER-ICA) was less impressive (Fig. 3b).

A number of additional tumour factors have been examined to determine whether they might aid discrimination between tamoxifen-sensitive and tamoxifen-resistant tumours, particularly in tumours with intermediate levels of oestrogen receptor (20-200 fmol/mg cytosol protein). However, progesterone receptor, EGF receptor, c-erbB2, microvessel count, Ki-S1, bcl-2, p53 and pS2 as measured by immunohistochemistry did not prove to be of value in this context (data not shown).

Changes in Ki-S1 and bcl-2 with treatment

The proliferation marker Ki-S1 [2] and the putative cell survival protein bcl-2 [3] have been measured by immunohistochemistry in tumours from elderly patients with ER-rich tumours before and after three months of treatment with tamoxifen. Changes in the proportion of tumour cells staining for both markers were observed and these have been categorised as described previously [4]. These are subdivided according to the clinical response in Table 2. The majority of responding tumours showed a decrease in Ki-S1 with treatment whereas most non-responding cancers displayed either no change or an increase in staining;

Table 2. Relationships between change in expression of Ki-S1, bcl-2 and response to primary tamoxifen therapy in 51 elderly women with breast cancer

(a) **Relationship with Ki-S1**

Immunohistochemical staining

	Decrease	No change/Increase
Responders	23	14
Non-responders	5	9

(b) **Relationship with bcl-2**

Immunohistochemical staining

	Decrease	No change/Increase
Responders	21	16
Non-responders	5	9

(c) **Relationship with concordant/discordant change**

	Concordant	Discordant
Responders	9	28
Non-responders	2	12

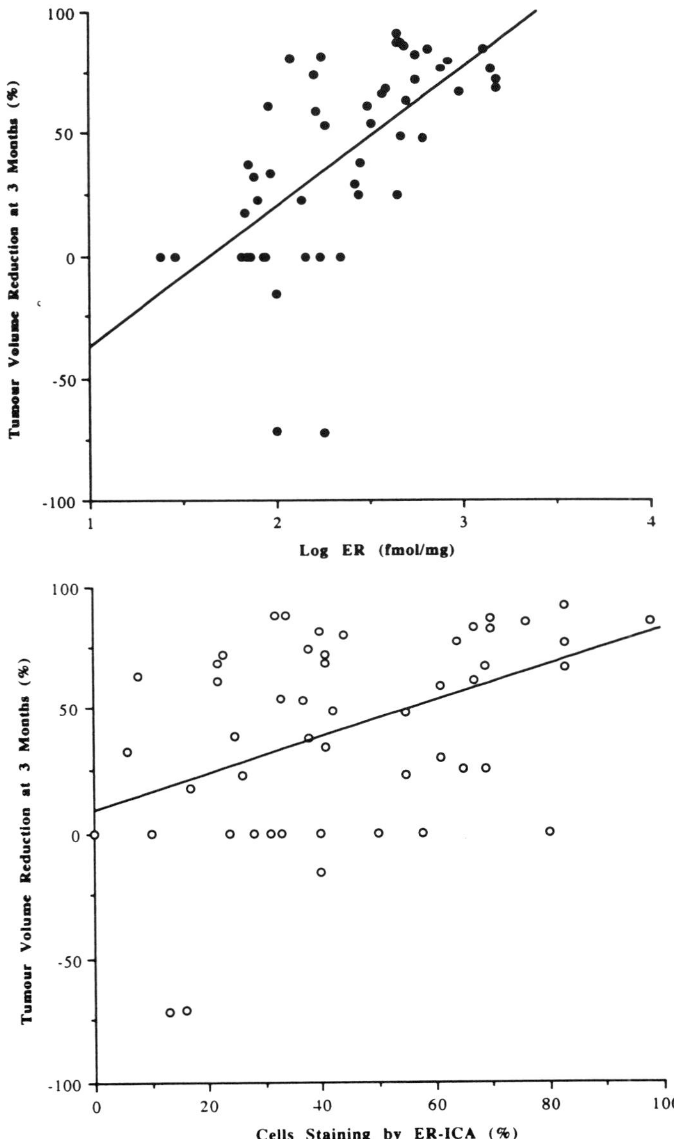

Fig. 3. Relationships between degree of tumour response and (a) oestrogen receptor values as assessed by ELISA (Abbott ER-EIA) on a biopsy and (b) oestrogen receptor values as assessed by ERICA on fine needle aspirates.

this difference was statistically significant between the groups. Changes in bcl-2 showed a similar pattern, with responding tumours tending to be associated with a decrease in staining and the reverse trend being observed in non-responding tumours. Although the different patterns of change in responding and non-responding tumours were similar for both Ki-S1 and bcl-2, individual tumours rarely showed concordant changes in the two markers, irrespective of tamoxifen-response status (Table 2c).

These patients now have five years of follow-up. The incidence of recurrent disease is higher among the 14 non-responding tumours (50%) than among the 37 responsive tumours (22%). Interestingly, however, the small cohort of eight patients who, although responding to treatment, failed to show a decrease in either Ki-S1 or bcl-2, had a recurrence rate identical to the non-responding tumours. It may be that residual high expression of Ki-S1/bcl-2 following successful therapy is a marker of a resistant and aggressive phenotype.

Neoadjuvant treatment with third-generation aromatase inhibitors

Recently, novel drugs have been developed which are able to inhibit the aromatase enzyme which catalyses the conversion of androgens into oestrogen potently and specifically. These agents include formestane, exemestane, anastrozole and letrozole [5-7]. Although they were piloted in advanced disease, the Edinburgh Unit has used the triazoles (anastrozole and letrozole) as primary systemic therapy. We have confirmed that in this setting letrozole markedly inhibits aromatase activity in the periphery and also that within the breast [8]. A consequence of the latter is that tumour endogenous oestrogens are markedly reduced on treatment [9]. It has therefore been of interest to examine the effects of treatment with these agents on the clinical volume and histopathology of the breast tumour. To do this, we have studied postmenopausal women with large (>3 cm) primary ER-rich breast cancers. All women had a tumour biopsy before entry to the study, three months' treatment with the aromatase inhibitor (during which time tumour volume was assessed clinically, by mammography and by ultrasound) followed by definitive breast surgery to remove residual tumour. In the case of anastrozole, patients were randomised to receive either 1 mg anastrozole daily (12 women) or 10 mg daily (11 women). The effects on tumour volume, as measured by ultrasound measurements, are shown in Table 3. The majority of women had a >50% decrease in tumour volume by three months and an example of tumour response is presented in Figure 4a. The median tumour reduction in size was 80% in the 1 mg group and 70% in the 10 mg group. Interestingly, although 17 of the patients at entry to study would have required a mastectomy to remove the primary tumour, after treatment with anastrozole 15 were suitable for breast-conserving surgery.

A similar group of patients have been treated with either 2.5 or 10 mg of letrozole; clinical responses are shown in Table 4. All but one patient experienced a clear reduction in tumour volume; an example of such a response is presented in Figure 4b. Fourteen of these patients would have required a mastecto-

Table 3. Clinical response in 23 women with large ER-rich breast cancers following primary systemic treatment with anastrozole (Arimidex)

	Number of patients	
	Arimidex 1mg/day	Arimidex 10mg/day
Lesions disappeared	0	0
>75% decrease*	8	4
50% - 75% decrease	3	3
<50% - 25% increase	1	4
>25% increase	0	0
Median reduction at 3 months	80.5%	69.6%

* % changes from baseline measurements at 3 months as assessed from ultrasound measurements of tumour volume

Table 4. Clinical and pathological responses following primary systemic treatment with letrozole (Femara) or with tamoxifen

	Letrozole	Tamoxifen
Clinical response		
Responders*	23	15
Non-responders	1	9
Total	24	24
Pathological response		
Complete	1	0
Microscopic residual	3	4
Partial	14	9
No change	6	11
Total	24	24

* At least 25% reduction in tumour volume at three months as assessed from ultrasound

my before treatment with letrozole, but after therapy all were managed by breast conservation. To put these observations into the context of other endocrine therapies, we have compared the letrozole patients with a similar group of women treated for three months with neoadjuvant tamoxifen over roughly the same time period (Table 4). The clinical response rate for tamoxifen was 63%

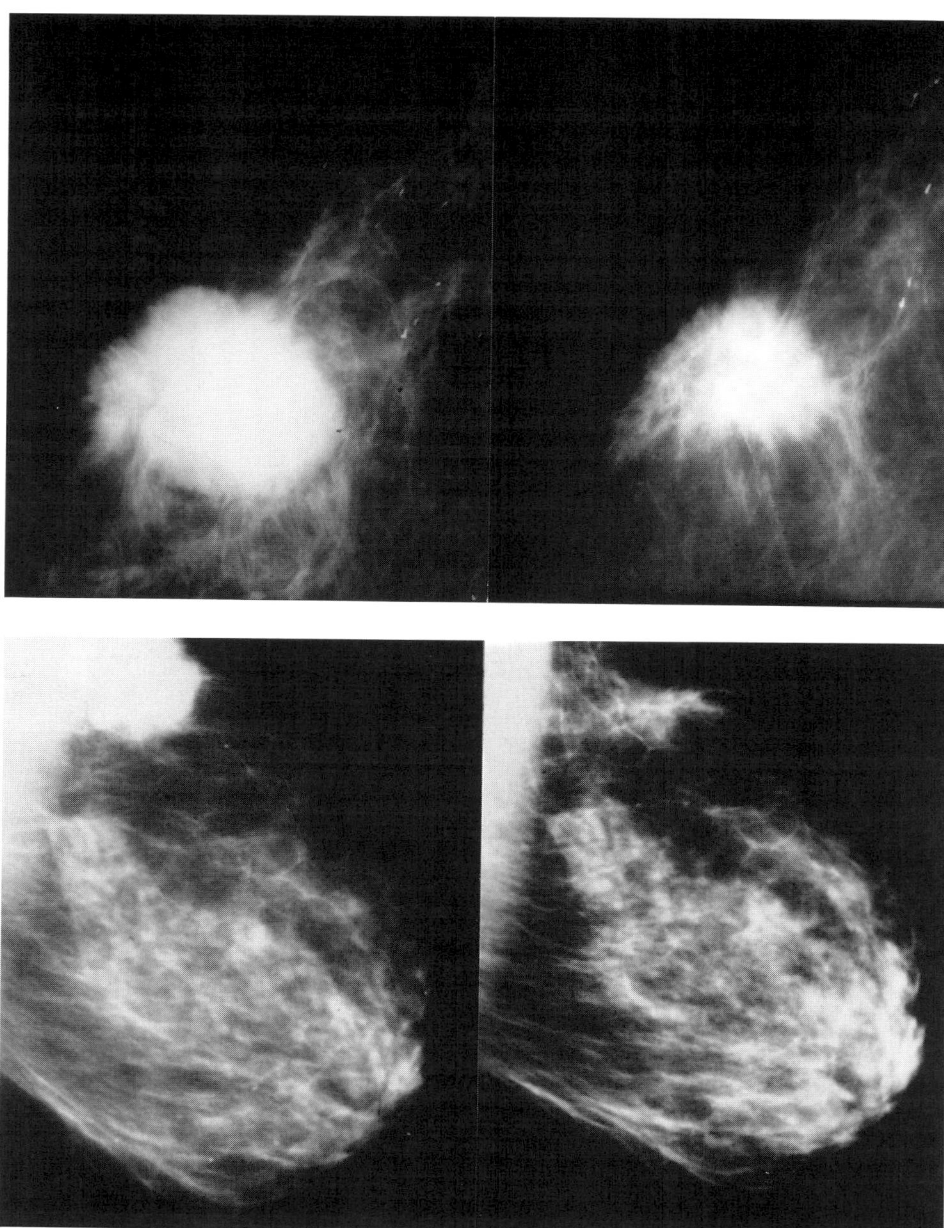

Fig. 4. Mammograms of the same breast before and after treatment either with anastrozole (top) or letrozole (bottom) showing clear resolution of the primary tumour with therapy.

(which is similar to our neoadjuvant tamoxifen experience in over 200 patients). This was substantially less than that observed with letrozole, where 96% of patients showed a tumour volume reduction of ≥25%. Pathological response was also compared and these results are also summarized in Table 4. Amongst the 24 patients treated with letrozole there was one complete pathological response, three cases with only minimal microscopic residual disease and 14 partial responses (either a clear decrease in tumour cellularity or an increase in fibrosis), representing a 75% response rate; the corresponding figure for tamoxifen was 54%. The proliferation marker Mib1 was also measured in sections from the same tumours. Letrozole-treatment was associated with a decrease in Mib1 in all cases (an example is shown in Fig. 5), whereas the pattern of change was less consistent with tamoxifen, only 18 of the 24 patients showing a decrease. This would be compatible with effects on histological grade: a change in grade characteristics was seen in both letrozole and tamoxifen series (10 cases), but the fall in grading score with letrozole was accounted for by a reduction in mitosis whereas an increase in tubule proportion was mainly responsible for the effect in tamoxifen-treated tumours. These results suggest that third-generation aromatase inhibitors are effective antitumour agents but their mechanism(s) of inducing response may differ from those of tamoxifen. This may have consequences for clinical management of the disease.

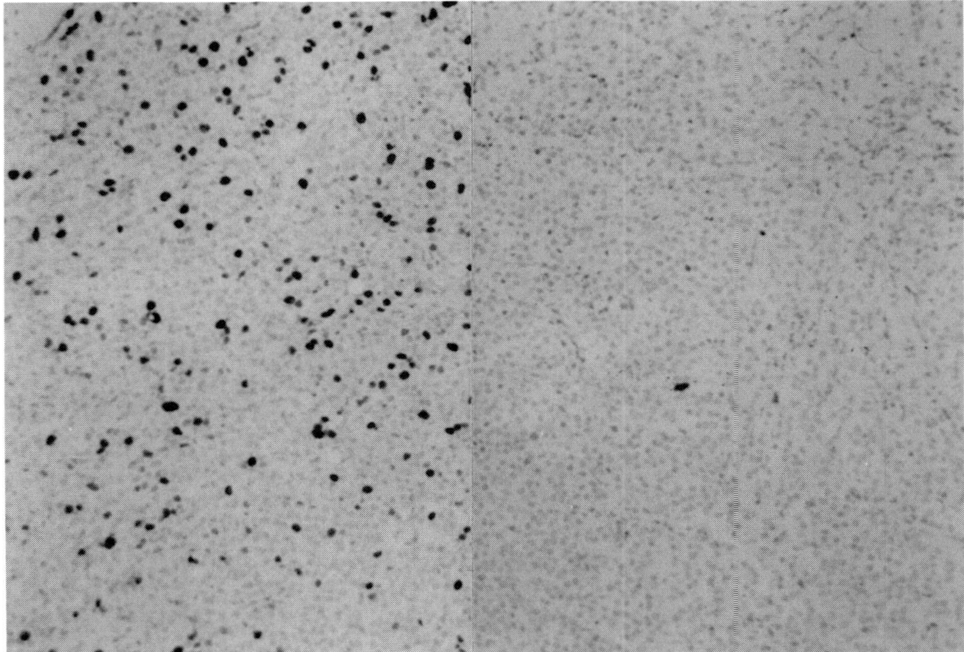

Fig. 5. Mib1 staining of the same tumour before and after treatment with three months' letrozole in a patient with breast cancer.

Summary and conclusions

The extensive experience of neoadjuvant endocrine therapy in Edinburgh has shown that in selected groups of women with large primary tumours or elderly patients the approach will produce clinical benefits in terms of (i) downstaging tumours so that more conservative breast surgery may be performed, and (ii) identifying endocrine-responsive tumours against those that are resistant, thus enabling rational decision-making concerning the continued use of endocrine agents in the adjuvant setting. Our results suggest that selection should include oestrogen receptor status, as responses are rarely observed in oestrogen receptor-poor tumours, irrespective of the type of endocrine treatment. On the other hand, in ER-rich tumours high response rates may be achieved. For example, in five different but overlapping series of women given neoadjuvant tamoxifen, the clinical response rates (as determined by at least a 25% reduction in tumour volume by ultrasound) ranged between 63 and 75% (median 71%); this response was achieved within three months.

Whilst we can identify groups of women with a low likelihood of response (ER-poor tumours) and high likelihood of response (ER-rich, >200 fmol/mg cytosol), prediction of response from initial tumour characteristics is not possible for many cancers. New markers are therefore still required and the option of monitoring changes in tumour biology which occur at very early time-points into treatment may be useful. Such studies are ongoing in several centres. Tumour measurements at later time-points in treatment may provide evidence of resistance to treatment; indeed, we have preliminary data to suggest that tumours which have responded to tamoxifen treatment but do not display a responsive phenotype in terms of changes in Ki-S1 and bcl-2 have high early recurrence rates, equivalent to those of tumours which have not responded. Finally, the approach of neoadjuvant therapy represents an important test-bed for determining the efficacy and mechanism of action of new endocrine agents. In this respect we have presented results which indicate that third-generation aromatase inhibitors such as anastrozole and letrozole are capable of producing profound clinical and pathological effects within breast cancers. These influences may be both more marked and different from those elicited by tamoxifen. The results merit more extensive studies including randomised trials. The final perspective is that the human tumour model described by Forrest et al. in 1986 [1] is delivering fundamental knowledge both in terms of clinical benefits and tumour biology; increased exploitation is urged and future results are eagerly awaited.

References

1   Forrest APM, Levack P, Chetty U et al. A human tumour model. The Lancet 1986; 2: 840-2
2   Kreipe H, Heidebrecht HJ, Hansen S et al. A new proliferation-associated nuclear antigen detectable in paraffin-embedded tissues by the monoclonal antibody Ki-S1. Am J Pathol 1993; 142: 3-9
3   Hockenbery D, Zutter M, Hickey W, Nahm M, Korsmeyer SJ. Bcl-2 protein is topographically restricted in tissues characterised by apoptotic cell death. Proc Natl Acad Sci USA 1991; 88: 6961-5
4   Keen JC, Dixon JM, Miller E et al. Expression of Ki-S1 and BCL-2 and the response to primary tamoxifen therapy in elderly patients with breast cancer. Breast Cancer Res Treat 1997; 44: 123-34
5   Lønning PE. Pharmacological profiles of exemestane and formestane, steroidal aromatase inhibitors used for treatment of postmenopausal breast cancer. Breast Cancer Res Treat 1998; 49: S45-S52
6   Plourde PV, Dyroff M, Dukes M. Arimidex® - A potent and selective 4th generation aromatase inhibitor. Breast Cancer Res Treat 1994; 30: 103-11
7   Smith IE, Norton A. Fadrozole and letrozole in advanced breast cancer: clinical and biochemical effects. Breast Cancer Res Treat 1998; 49: S67-S71
8   Miller WR. Biology of aromatase inhibitors: pharmacology/endocrinology within the breast. Endocrine Related Cancer 1999 (in press)
9   Miller WR, Telford J, Love C et al. Effects of letrozole as primary medical therapy on in situ oestrogen synthesis and endogenous oestrogen levels within the breast. The Breast 1998; 7: 273-6

ESO Scientific Updates, Vol. 4
Primary Medical Therapy for Breast Cancer
A. Howell and M. Dowsett, editors
© 1999 Elsevier Science B.V. All rights reserved

New Approaches in Molecular Tumour Biology

Henri Magdelénat

Department of Translational Research and Technology Transfer, Institut Curie, Paris,
France. Receptor and Biomarker Study Group, EORTC

Introduction

As with other tumour types, such as osteosarcomas and head and neck cancers,
primary medical treatment (PMT) – also referred to as neoadjuvant or preoperative systemic therapy – has become standard practice for locally advanced
breast cancer. The rationale for PMT is based on three hypotheses, which are
either biological or clinical:

- PMT creates less favourable growth kinetics for micrometastases at the time
  of surgery
- PMT allows to assess tumour response *in vivo*, and thus drug resistance
- PMT should increase the rate of breast conservation.

However, PMT also has potential limitations, for example, it may allow
the tumour to progress to an inoperable stage, it may imply overtreatment of a
number of patients, and it may result in loss of pathological and biological
prognostic factors.

From the few clinical trials evaluated so far it appears that PMT presents
acceptable safety and results in a slight but favourable increase in breast conservation, thus offering an alternative to primary surgical locoregional treatment. However, analysis of the available data suggests that the real benefit
(i.e. in terms of disease-free and overall survival) is seen only in patients who
achieve a pathological complete remission (pCR) [1,2]. It is therefore very important to detect early – ideally pretreatment – prognosticators of response to
PMT besides prognosticators of DFS and OS.

PMT offers a unique opportunity to assess the value of biological markers in
predicting clinical response and, even more important for the future, to study
the influence of treatment on the biological response (and adaptation) of the
tumour during the whole period before tumour excision.

Address for correspondence: H. Magdelénat, Laboratoire de Transfert, Institut Curie,
26 rue d'Ulm, 75248 Paris Cedex 05, France. Tel.: +33-1-44324270, fax: +33-1-44324073,
e-mail: henri.magdelenat@curie.fr

Tumour sampling

In the context of PMT, biological investigations are hampered by the availability of only a limited amount of tumour tissue. There are two ways to obtain tissue samples (Fig. 1):

1) cytological fine needle sampling (FNS), preferably without aspiration in order to avoid blood contamination. This technique is particularly suitable for biochemical or molecular analysis, for the following reasons [3,4]:
* immediate evaluation of cell density
* homogeneity >90% due to absence of stromal or blood cells
* representation of all malignant clones in the tumour (multidirectional)
* immediate freezing of the sample
* painless and repeatable during PMT.

2) Since microbiopsies (core biopsies) and trucuts provide tiny histological specimens (<10 mg) that are not representative of the whole tumour, drill biopsies [5] should be preferred. This technique allows to obtain substantial histological material (20-80 mg) throughout the tumour mass, albeit with a variable stromal component. It requires local anaesthesia and is not easily repeatable.

Both types of tumour samples (FNS and drill biopsies) should be frozen immediately in liquid nitrogen for analysis of protein (ER, PgR, TK, etc.) or mRNA gene expression (see below). Analysis of genetic alterations at DNA level (molecular biology or FISH) is possible on fixed (AFA) sections of drill biopsies or of FNS smears.

Molecular biology

Biochemical analysis (RIA, ELISA, enzymatic assays) allows the analysis of very few – not more than three – biological parameters on FNS or microbiopsies, and requires careful subcellular cell fractionation. Immunohistochemistry may give more biological information but is limited by the scarce availability of reproducible and specific antibodies and by the difficulty of reproducible and quantitative detection.

In contrast, the specificity and sensitivity of molecular biology, in particular the amplification of target sequences by polymerase chain reaction (PCR), allow, even on such small samples, the analysis of a significant set of biological parameters (up to 30 for a FNS) without limitations for reagents (synthetic oligonucleotides). It thus offers great potential for monitoring tumour biology in the context of PMT.

In order to analyse gene expression at the mRNA level by PCR, mRNA first has to be transcribed into complementary DNA (cDNA) by reverse transcription (RT). Genetic alterations (such as gene amplification, deletion, mutation, etc.) can be readily assessed on genomic DNA by PCR. It is recommended to transcribe

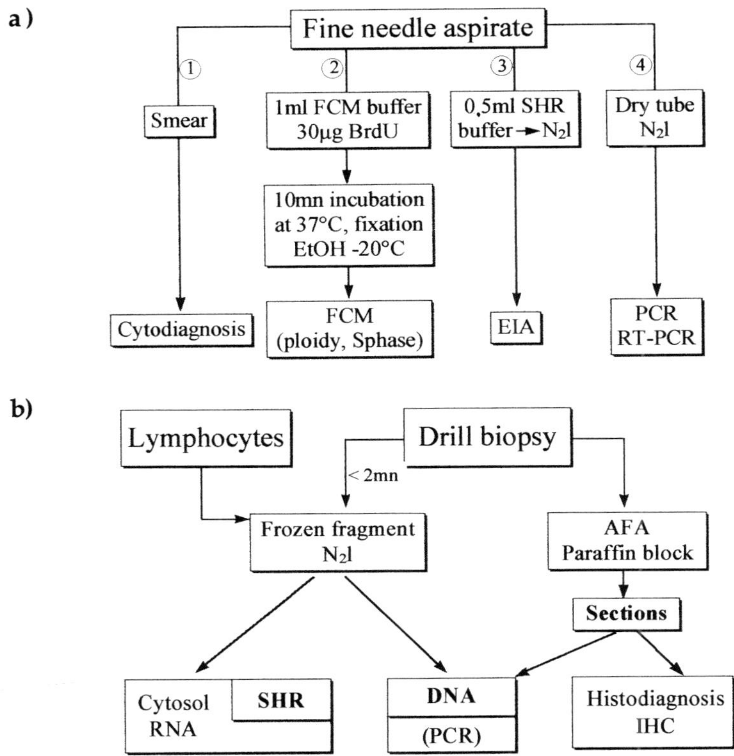

Fig. 1. Collection and distribution of tumour samples. a) Fine needle aspirate; b) drill or core biopsy.

all mRNAs present in the tumour cells in order to allow multiparametric analysis. This is achieved by non-specific reverse transcription with random hexamers as primers.

Measurement of gene expression

Semiquantitative RT-PCR

mdr1: mdr1 gene expression has been measured by semiquantitative RT-PCR on retrotranscribed mRNA extracted from fine needle samples obtained for the monitoring of PMT in breast cancer [6,7].

The co-amplification of a "reference cDNA" (b_2 microglobulin or b_2m) with mdr1 cDNA led to a relative quantification of mdr1 gene expression. This assay was used to evaluate the predictive value of mdr1 and its evolution during the first cycle of chemotherapy [6]. Eighty-eight patients with untreated lesions (T2 >3 cm, T3, M0) were randomised between four cycles of CAF (C, cyclophosphamide; A, doxorubicin; F, fluorouracil) and four cycles of CTF (T, thiotepa); doxorubicin was administered on day 1 and 8 of each cycle. The mdr1 gene was expressed in 25% of the 73 evaluable patients. Pretreatment expression was weakly predictive of resistance in the FAC arm (predictive value 66%) but not in the FTC arm. However, in both arms an increase in mdr1 gene expression between day 0 and day 8 of the first cycle of chemotherapy invariably resulted in treatment failure (predictive value 100%). In a subsequent trial the full dose of doxorubicin was administered on day 1 and the predictive value of mdr1 expression (pretreatment or on day 8) was lost. This strongly suggests that the administration of doxorubicin after induction of mdr1 decreases its therapeutic efficacy.

In the long term, mdr1 mRNA expression showed prognostic value in univariate and multivariate analysis (Cox model). However, this was much weaker than the prognostic value of S-phase for DFS and OS [7].

The fact that in the FTC arm an increase in mdr1 mRNA was frequently observed, although the intracellullar uptake of none of the three FTC drugs is known to be controlled by gP170 (mdr1 protein), suggests that multidrug resistance is not dependent on a single effector. Most probably a set of various drug resistance-related genes are simultaneously involved. Therefore a multiparametric analysis of inducible drug resistance genes (e.g. MRP, LRP, GSTπ) might improve early prediction of response.

Although simple in its principle, semiquantitative PCR is poorly reproducible and analyses of different parameters, currently under investigation in new PMT trials, are being performed with improved quantitative methods (see below). The merit of the initial studies was to prove that useful medical information can be obtained from the analysis of a single analyte, i.e. total RNA.

Quantitative PCR

Two approaches can be used to improve the quantitative performance of (RT) PCR.

Competitive PCR [8] involves the simultaneous amplification of not only both the target gene and the reference gene, but also that of a known amount of slightly modified cDNA copies (mimics) of the target and the reference genes. Thus, the absolute number of target cDNA in the sample can be accurately calculated. This method is more accurate and reproducible but requires the construction of modified nucleotide sequences and high resolution analysis of PCR fragments by capillary electrophoresis or gel electrophoresis, both expensive techniques. It has been successfully applied to the analysis of various cytokines expressed in tumour tissues [9].

We have applied competitive RT-PCR to the assay of ER and PgR mRNA expression in surgical samples. A close correlation was found between RT-PCR and protein expression (ER and PgR EIA) (Fig. 2). Although this technology is

PgR

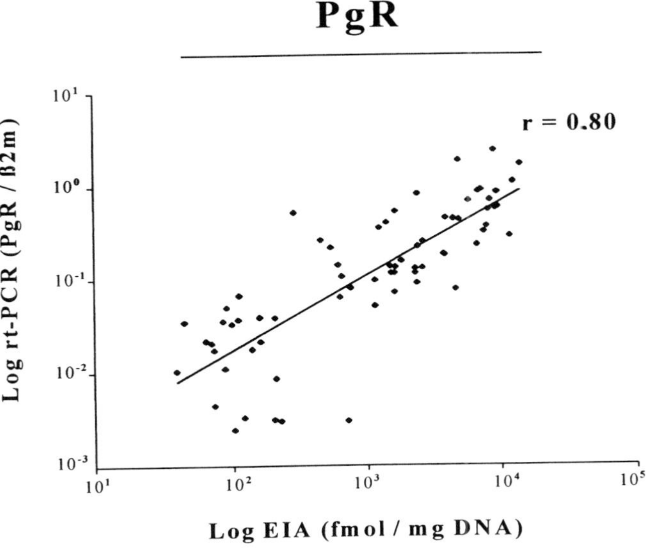

Fig. 2. Progesterone receptor: correlation between protein expression (EIA) and mRNA expression (RT-PCR).

not widely employed for ER and PgR due to the present ease of use of immuno-histochemistry or EIA in small biopsy specimens, it proved that, at least for some parameters like ER or PgR, mRNA quantitation correlates with quantitative protein expression. Thus, the assay of ER and PgR mRNA by easier methods (see below) might be valuable in the future to determine the receptor status together with other parameters.

We have used competitive PCR also to measure HER/neu (c-erbB2) gene amplification on AFA fixed sections of drill biopsies (Fig. 3) [10]. Three 10 mm sections of the drill biopsies proved to be sufficient for the assay. We have constructed a single plasmid (pTag) harbouring one modified sequence (4bp deletion) of each HER/neu and a reference gene (GAPDH). Thus the average copy number of the tumour sample can be accurately determined, with discrimination between clearly amplified samples (>4 HER/neu copies per diploid genome) and non-amplified samples (≤2 copies). The ambiguity between two and four copies is mainly due to imprecision in the estimation of the stromal contribution to tumour cellularity.

Drill biopsy specimens from 81 patients treated by PMT (AC vs AT) at the Institut Curie were assayed in parallel for HER/neu amplification and protein expression (immunohistochemical staining with CB11 MAb [15]). Five samples (6%) could not be analysed due to a low DNA extraction yield, and seven (9%) with apparently no amplification were considered as non-informative since the histological percentage of tumour cells was less than 20%. Twenty-two samples (27%) displayed amplification and 47 (57%) did not. Interestingly, amplifica-

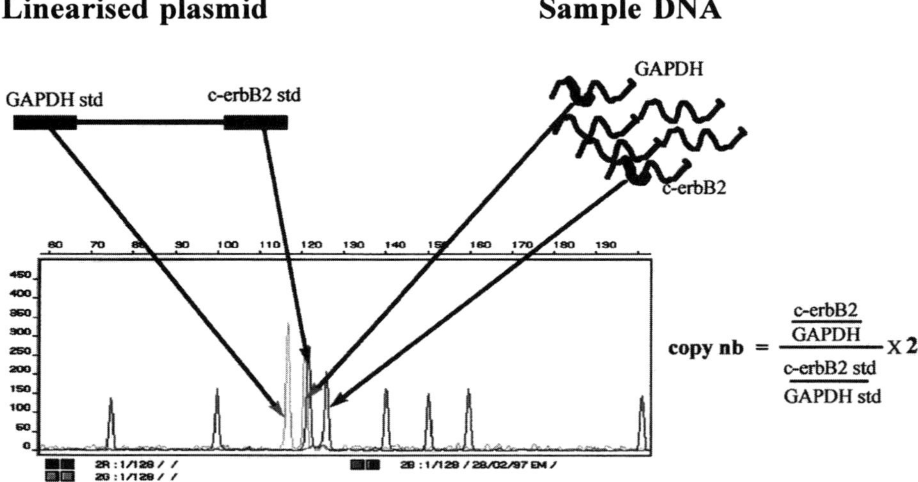

$$\text{copy nb} = \frac{\dfrac{\text{c-erbB2}}{\text{GAPDH}}}{\dfrac{\text{c-erbB2 std}}{\text{GAPDH std}}} \times 2$$

Fig. 3. Principle of competitive PCR applied to HER/neu amplification assay. Colour display allows identification of all peaks.

tion and overexpression were correlated, except in six amplified cases with low HER/neu expression. Analysis of response and outcome of patients will tell us more about the respective value of these assays.

In conclusion, gene amplification can be accurately measured in tumour drill biopsies. However, histological heterogeneity remains a limitation in quantitative molecular biology. Image analysis, microdissection or FISH (fluorescence *in situ* hybridization) may circumvent this problem.

Real-time PCR

With this method [11] an internal probe harbouring a reporter fluorophore (R) and a quencher (Q) is present during the amplification reaction. In its native state the probe does not fluorescence due to the proximity of the quencher. During strand replication the reporter fluorophore is cleaved by the polymerase 5' nucleotidase activity and the released fluorescence is detected in real time (Fig. 4).

Real-time PCR offers significant advantages for the accurate measurement of the level of DNA (or cDNA) sequences present in a sample:
- extremely good reproducibility of the assay endpoint, i.e. the calculated thermal cycle, when the fluorescence diverges from the background (Ct).
- amplification and detection in the same tube, reducing the risk of contamination. This risk is even decreased by enzymatic digestion (UNG) of PCR fragments. This is particularly important for routine clinical assays or when analysing micrometastases by (RT) PCR.
- high throughput (analysis of 96 samples completed in 3 hours).

REAL TIME DETECTION PCR

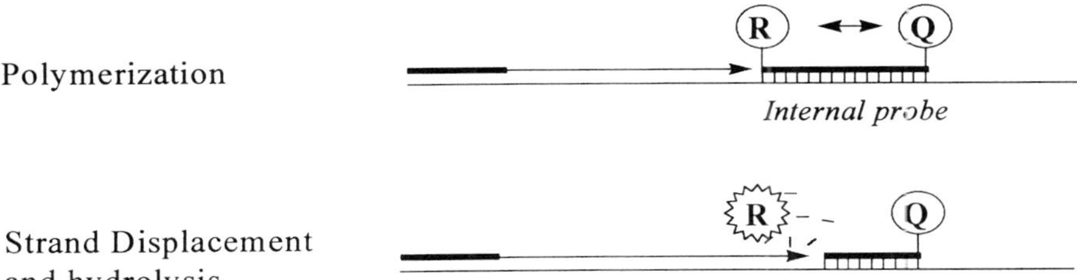

Fig. 4. Principle of real-time PCR. During the extension phase, the reporter dye R from the probe is released and separated from the quencher dye Q, resulting in increasing fluorescence of the reporter.

There is still a problem for duplex analysis, so the reference gene has to be analysed separately. However, the reproducibility is so good that this is not the major source of variation for RT-PCR.

We, and an increasing number of groups, are currently developing real-time PCR or RT-PCR assays. For instance, the quantitation of mdr1 gene expression and its reproducibility has been greatly increased by real-time RT-PCR. Standard curves using dilutions of a reference ovarian cell line (CEM) are now highly reproducible, with interassay coefficients of variation lower than 10%.

Although the number of biological parameters which can be assayed by this method is limited by the amount of total RNA extractable from FNS or microbiopsies, it is not less than 20. Some interesting biological parameters are listed in Table 1.

Table 1. Biological parameters and targets

Endocrine therapy	Chemo-therapy	Metastasis	Apoptosis	Immunology
ER	mdr1	uPA	bax	IL-x
PgR	mrp	PAI1	bcl-2	
Ncor	GSTπ	uPAR	caspase x	
SRC1	TK	MMP	fas	
Aromatase	TS	Cath-D	NFkB	
EGFR		FGF-R	p53	
erbB2	raf1 kin	VEGF	mdm2	
IGF1R		angiopoietin	SMase	
		TIE2	p300	

Thymidine kinase (TK) and thymidylate synthase (TS)

Tumour proliferation rate (S-phase) and proliferation-associated markers (Ki67) are proven prognosticators of response to chemotherapy and strong prognostic factors [7,12-14]. In this respect it is interesting to study those biological parameters related to proliferation that are, in addition, the targets of drugs currently used in PMT. TK and TS have such features, being directly involved in the mechanisms of action of antimetabolites such as MTX and 5FU [15-17]. TK is able to bypass the inhibition of DNA synthesis by TS inhibitors. The Receptor Biomarker Study Group of the EORTC is currently developing the assays of TK and TS by real-time RT-PCR (P.M. Martin, Marseille) in order to confirm the relation between TK level and resistance to TS inhibitors, and demonstrate that patients with high TK benefit from drugs related to other targets (e.g. taxanes) in an EORTC primary chemotherapy trial comparing 5FU intensification to taxane (Protocol New 10921).

For the study of the influence of tumour biology on response to PMT we believe it is most appropriate to primarily investigate those biological parameters that are known to interact with new drugs. Thus, the VEGF mRNA assay is also being developed in view of clinical trials with inhibitors of angiogenesis.

Influence of treatment on tumour biology

Useful information has been derived from the study of the influence of treatment on tumour biology by sequential analysis of tumour samples. The study of the variations of steroid hormone receptors during primary endocrine and/or chemotherapy [18-20] has led to a better understanding of tumour resistance and second-line response. The sequential study of S-phase [20] and mdr1 [6] expression during PMT has allowed to unravel the *in vivo* effects of different drugs.

From these studies, as well as from cytogenetic analyses [21], the biology of breast cancer appears to be very complex, which stresses the need for multiparametric biological information. Whole genome approaches are in progress to analyse this complexity.

Pharmacogenomics

New tools, such as microarrays (or biochips) or microfluidic devices, already allow the simultaneous analysis of the expression of several thousands of genes [22,23] of known or even unknown function. This approach can be completed by the analysis of the "proteome", i.e. the analysis by 2D electrophoresis and mass spectrometry of thousands of differentially expressed proteins.

At the present time, the cost of such analyses and the need for sophisticated data analysis systems preclude extensive use of this technology for individual patients. However, it is to be hoped that, either from experimental models or from selected clinical situations, the most informative biological parameters

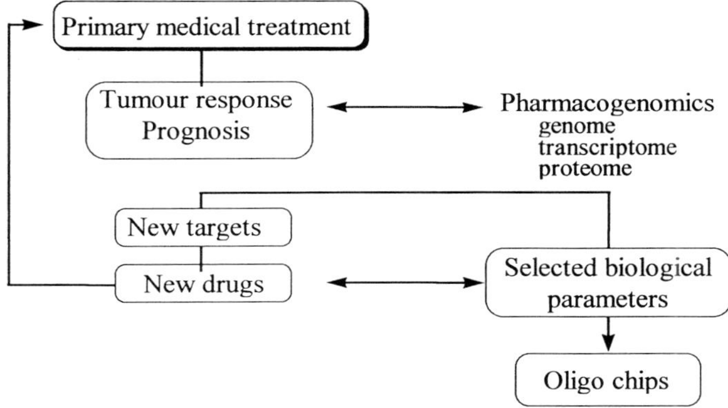

Fig. 5. Directions for the future.

will be selected. These selected indicators will then be analysed on smaller, dedicated "minichips" for the management of PMT. In addition, pharmacogenomics is expected to define new biological targets and orient the development of new drugs (Fig. 5).

The search for surrogate endpoints

The control of micrometastases present before treatment or released during surgery is a major goal of PMT. Thus, the detection and characterisation of malignant cells in peripheral blood and/or in bone marrow constitutes a biological staging parameter that is worth evaluating.

Surgery is known to release tumour cells in the circulation. The detection of tumour cells in peripheral blood or bone marrow can be achieved directly by (RT) PCR, provided a genetic or phenotypic trait characterises malignant clones. Unfortunately, there is no specific trait for breast cancer and the detection is based on the expression of cytokeratins (CK 19) and mucins (MUC1). We have developed an RT-PCR-based detection assay which combines immuno-magnetic separation of mammary cells with beads coated with anti Ber EP4 antibody protein (mammary cell selective adhesion glycoprotein) (Dynal, Oslo, Norway), and real-time RT-PCR of MUC1 mRNA. In these conditions, the detection appears very sensitive (<1 cell per ml of peripheral blood) and specific (no false positives in healthy subjets and in patients with benign tumours).

Circulating cells can theoretically be further characterized by the expression of candidate mRNA associated with the metastatic phenotype (uPA receptor, mts1, etc.) by (RT) PCR or on gene expression microarrays. Molecular biology allows the study of phenotypic profiles at the level of single cells.

Alternatively, and apparently more efficiently in bone marrow, micrometastases can be detected by immunocytofluorescence of cytospinned or membrane-filtered samples with anti-cytokeratin antibodies such as AB45B/B3 [24]. Individual cytokeratin-positive cells can be further characterized by double immunochemical staining (e.g. for uPAR) or FISH. Individual cells can also be transferred by microdissection from the cytospinned slides or from membranes directly into a tube where they can be analysed by (RT) PCR for genotypic or phenotypic processes [25].

Many of these new methodologies have to be validated both technically and clinically but they represent invaluable approaches for investigating the complex and probably individual relationship between the biology of breast tumours and their response to various modalities of treatment.

Conclusion

In order to optimise PMT of breast cancer, a better understanding of tumour biology is required. New approaches, many of them by molecular biology technology, will make it possible to collect much more biological information than in the past. The Receptor and Biomarker Study Group of the EORTC, with a long tradition of quality assurance in tumour biology, has organised a task force for the validation of methods for the detection and characterisation of micro-metastases, which should serve the monitoring of PMT efficacy.

Acknowledgements

Many of the data discussed in this article were generated by or with the help of colleagues from the Institut Curie: Prof. P. Pouillart, Dr V. Dieras and Dr J.Y. Pierga (Medical Oncology), Dr X. Sastre-Garau (Pathology), Dr P. Vielh (Cytopathology), Dr P. de Cremoux and Dr Y. Remvikos (Physiopathology), and S. Chevillard (Department of Translational Research).

References

1   Fisher B, Bryant J, Wolmark N et al. Effect of preoperative chemotherapy on the outcome of women with operable breast cancer (NSABP) B-18. J Clin Oncol 1998; 16: 2672-85
2   Scholl SM, Pierga JY, Asselain B et al. Breast tumour response to primary chemotherapy predicts local and distant control as well as survival. Eur J Cancer 1995; 31A: 1969-75
3   Zajdela A, Zilhardt P, Voilmot N. Cytological diagnosis by fine needle sampling without aspiration. Cancer 1987; 59: 1201-5
4   Magdelénat H, Lainé-Bidron C, Merle S, Zajdela A. Estrogen and progestin receptor assays in fine needle aspirates of breast cancer. Eur J Clin Oncol 1987; 23: 425-31
5   Magdelénat H. Forage biopsie et cytoponction pour la détermination des récepteurs hormonaux. Path Biol 1985; 31: 755-60
6   Chevillard S, Pouillart P, Beldjord C et al. Sequential assessment of multidrug resistance phenotype and measurement of S-phase fraction as predictive markers of breast cancer response to neoadjuvant chemotherapy. Cancer 1996; 77: 292-9

7   Chevillard S, Lebeau J, Pouillart P et al. Biological and clinical significance of concurrent p53 gene alterations, mdr1 gene expression and S-phase fraction analyses in breast cancer patients treated with primary chemotherapy or radiotherapy. Clin Cancer Res 1997; 3: 24

8   Raeymaekers L. Quantitative PCR: theoretical considerations with practical implications. Anal Biochem 1993; 214: 582-5

9   Tartour E, Gey A, Sastre-Garau X et al. Prognostic value of intratumoral IFNγ messenger RNA expression in invasive cervical carcinoma. JNCI 1998; 90: 287-94

10   de Cremoux P, Martin EC, Vincent-Salomon A et al. Quantitative PCR analysis of c-erbB2 gene amplification and comparison with p185 expression in breast cancer drill biopsies. Int J Cancer 1999 (in press).

11   Bieche I, Olivi M, Champeme MH, Vidaud D, Lidereau R, Vidaud M. Novel approach to quantitative polymerase chain reaction using real-time detection of gene amplification in breast cancer. Int J Cancer 1998; 78(5): 661-6

12   Remvikos Y, Mosseri V, Zajdela A et al. Prognostic value of S-phase fraction of breast cancers treated by primary radiotherapy or neoadjuvant chemotherapy. Ann NY Acad Sci 1993; 698: 193-203

13   Pierga JY, Leroyer A, Vielh P et al. Long term prognostic value of growth fraction determination by Ki67 immunostaining in primary operable breast cancer. Breast Cancer Res Treat 1996; 37(1); 57-64

14   Remvikos Y, Mosseri V, Asselain B et al. S-phase fractions of breast cancer predict overall and post relapse survival. Eur J Cancer 1997; 33(4): 581-5

15   Rozan S, Vincent-Salomon A, Zafrani B et al. No significant predictive value of c-erbB2 or p53 expression regarding sensitivity to primary chemotherapy or radiotherapy in breast cancer. Int J Cancer 1998; 79(1): 27-33

16   Romain S, Martin PM, Klijn JG et al. DNA synthesis enzyme activity: a biological tool useful for predicting anti-metabolic drug sensitivity in breast cancer? Int J Cancer 1997; 74(2): 156-61

17   Leichman CG, Lenz HJ, Leichman L et al. Quantitation of intratumoral TS expression predicts disseminated colorectal cancer response and resistance to protracted infusion fluorouracil and weekly leucovorin. J Clin Oncol 1997; 15: 3223-9

18   Magdelénat H, Merle S, Zajdela A. Enzyme immunoassay of estrogen receptors in fine needle aspirates of breast tumours. Cancer Res 1986; 46 (Suppl): 4265-7

19   Jouve M, Palangié T, Dorval T et al. Evolution de la concentration en récepteurs hormonaux sous chimiothérapie cytotoxique. Bull Cancer 1986; 73(3): 271-78

20   Remvikos Y, Jouve M, Beuzeboc P et al. Cell cycle modifications of breast cancers during neoadjuvant chemotherapy: a flow cytometry study on fine needle aspirates. Eur J Cancer 1993; 29A(13): 1843-8

21   Magdelénat H, Gerbault-Seureau M, Lainé-Bidron C et al. Genetic evolution of breast cancer, II. Relationship with estrogen and progesterone receptor expression. Breast Cancer Res Treat 1992; 22: 119-27

22   Lockhart D, Dong H, Byrne MC et al. Expression monitoring hybridization to high-density oligonucleotide arrays. Nature Biotech 1996; 14: 1675-80

23   De Risi J, Penland L, Brown PO et al. Use of cDNA microarray to analyse gene expression patterns in human cancer. Nature Genetics 1996; 14: 457-60

24   Kvalheim G. Diagnosis of minimal residual disease in bone marrow and blood in cancer patients. Acta Oncologica 1998; 37: 456-62

25   Bernsen MR, Dijkman HB, de Vries E et al. Identification of multiple RNA and DNA sequences from small tissue samples isolated by laser assisted microdissection. Laboratory Invest 1998; 78(10): 1267-73

ESO Scientific Updates, Vol. 4
Primary Medical Therapy for Breast Cancer
A. Howell and M. Dowsett, editors
© 1999 Elsevier Science B.V. All rights reserved

Biological Studies in Primary Medical Therapy of Breast Cancer: The Royal Marsden Hospital Experience

M. Dowsett, I.E. Smith, T.J. Powles, J. Salter, P.A. Ellis[1], S.R.D. Johnston, A. Makris[2], P. Mainwaring, R.K. Gregory, C. Archer, J. Chang[3] and L. Assersohn

Academic Department of Biochemistry and Department of Medicine, Royal Marsden Hospital, London and Sutton, United Kingdom

Current addresses: [1]Guys-Kings-St. Thomas Cancer Centre, London; [2]Mount Vernon Hospital, Middlesex, U.K.; [3]National University Hospital, Singapore

Introduction

The unique opportunity for studying the biology of breast cancer during therapy which is afforded by the scenario of primary medical therapy (PMT) has been recognised for many years [1]. While studies of prognosis in relation to biological and pathological characteristics of breast tumours are widespread, they are in many cases of dubious value: there is general acknowledgement that the discovery of predictive factors, i.e. markers which are indicative of response to or benefit from a specific therapeutic manoeuvre, would be of much greater value. PMT is well suited to address this issue, since biological measurements can be made in the same tumour in which clinical response occurs, and this response is more readily measured in the primary lesion than in metastatic sites. Many "bioclinical" studies have been conducted to identify predictive markers in adjuvant therapy or in advanced disease. However, in adjuvant therapy, since patients are clinically disease-free post-surgery, it is not possible to measure the *response* of an individual patient. In advanced disease biomarkers are generally measured in the primary lesion and response in metastases, such that the response is temporally, topographically and possibly biologically separated from the biomarker measurements.

The majority of studies on PMT have assessed only pre-treatment markers but sequential measurements in multiple samples during therapy may be at least as valuable. The changes noted may be predictive of response and in some cases, e.g. with changes in proliferation and apoptosis, the measurements may be intimately related to growth changes, such that these might be valid intermediate indices of response.

Address for correspondence: M. Dowsett, Academic Department of Biochemistry, The Royal Marsden Hospital, Fulham Road, London SW3 6JJ, United Kingdom. Tel.: +44-171-8082887, fax +44-171-3763918, e-mail: mitch@icr.ac.uk

Additionally, although primary medical therapy is generally associated with impressive response rates, pathological complete responses are infrequent. Studies of the residual tissue after the completion of medical therapy or at the time of maximal response should provide data on mechanisms of response and resistance. A straightforward view might be that studies of such residual cell populations should be our highest priority, since it is these populations which are the threat to the patients' welfare.

At the Royal Marsden Hospital we have conducted several clinical trials during the last decade (Table 1) and a programme of biological research as an integral component of them. During this time we have performed a series of validation studies which have helped to assess the variability of analyses, and thus the degree of change needed to be seen in an individual patient for it to be deemed significant. Our most recent data have focused on changes in proliferation and apoptosis; the validation studies relevant to these are discussed below.

Sampling techniques, advantages and disadvantages

We have employed core-cut biopsies and fine needle aspirates (FNAs) as sampling techniques for obtaining pre-treatment and on-treatment tumour tissue.

FNAs can, if conducted with care, be taken at frequent intervals (every few

Table 1. Clinical trials of primary medical therapy (PMT) providing biological material for analysis at the Royal Marsden Hospital. Analyses have also been conducted on patients given PMT outside of the trial setting.

Trial design	Drugs	Study period	No. patients
Randomised PMT vs Surgery	Mitoxantrone, methotrexate, tamoxifen	1989/1995	300
	Tamoxifen	1994/1996	40
Non-randomised PMT	Cyclophosphamide, methotrexate, 5-fluorouracil	1985/1990	64
	Epirubicin, cisplatin, 5-fluorouracil (ECF)	1990/1992	50
	ECF (+ tamoxifen) vs adriamycin, cyclophosphamide, tamoxifen	1993/1998	180

days) without undue distress to the patient. The number of cells obtained can vary substantially but may be >10^6. The cell suspension is particularly well suited to automated analytical techniques such as flow cytometry, but most of our analyses have been conducted on cytospins which, in the best cases, can yield several thousand cells/slide. Our early experience with FNAs demonstrated that multiple markers could be measured on a single FNA with generally good concordance with the same markers assessed by histology [2,3]. For example, 91.5% concordance was seen for oestrogen receptor (ER) when evaluated as ER$^+$ or ER$^-$. It was also shown that statistically significant correlations existed between ER and either PgR, bcl-2 or p53 (r = 0.61, 0.30, and -0.39, respectively), between p53 and S-phase fraction (SPF) or Ki67 (r = 0.33 and 0.40, respectively) and between Ki67 and S-phase (r = 0.56) [4]. This significant correlation between the two proliferation indices has not been reported by all groups, but was confirmed by our observation of a strong correlation between SPF in FNAs and Ki67 (measured as Mib1) in sections (rho = 0.59, n = 75, p <0.0001) [5]. It was notable, however, that SPF was not measurable in 31/164 (20%) aspirates either because of inadequate cellularity or overlapping peaks on DNA histogram [2].

A disadvantage of FNAs is that they do not allow invasive disease to be distinguished from *in situ* lesions on morphological grounds. However, in the near future advances in molecular pathology may allow analysis of a panel of markers to discriminate between the two.

Measurements of apoptosis have become a key element of our studies of response and resistance to PMT. However, the low number of apoptotic cells, even in treated tumours, makes the measurements laborious: normally ≥3000 cells need to be scored for sufficient statistical confidence. We have therefore attempted to automate our analyses of apoptosis by performing the TUNEL assay on cells taken by FNA, using flow cytometry for analysis [6]. In a pilot study of 12 patients we observed a significant correlation (p = 0.03) between the automated methodology and our standard methodology on sections. Further experience, however, has revealed two substantial difficulties with this technique: (i) the cutoff taken to define apoptotic and non-apoptotic cells without visual confirmation is unreliable; (ii) the TUNEL assay also stains fragmented DNA in areas of necrosis; this would usually be avoided in scoring apoptosis on sections but cannot be discriminated by flow cytometric approaches.

Core-cuts have the advantage of retaining the epithelial-stromal architecture of the tumour. In most of our studies a 14-gauge needle is used to provide a core which is c. 1.5 cm long by c. 2 mm diameter and weighs 20-30 mg. Each histological section through a highly cellular core can reveal >25,000 cells. Large numbers of sections from the same core can be available. The local trauma which may be caused, however, does not allow core-cuts to be made at frequent intervals.

Variability of analysis

The focus of our work on changes in proliferation and apoptosis has led us to evaluate the precision of the measurement of proliferation and apoptosis. Figure 1(a) and (b) show the reproducibility of measurements of Ki67 (Mib1) and apoptotic index (AI), respectively, as found in pairs of core-cuts taken immediately after one another from the same tumour. For Ki67 and AI the mean difference was 33% and 38%, respectively, and the standard deviation of the difference was 16% and 22%, respectively. In essence, for a pair of results to be considered significantly different from one another there needs to be a >50% difference between them [7].

A slightly different approach was taken to estimate the reproducibility of S-phase measurements; in this case the samples were taken 14 days apart but with no intervening treatment. The values of 25 pairs were strongly correlated, with no systematic difference between the first and second samples. This observation indicates that there are no significant alterations to SPF as a result of taking an earlier aspirate [3]. Similar data have also been derived indicating no significant change in ER, PgR, Ki67, p53 and bcl-2 in FNAs [8].

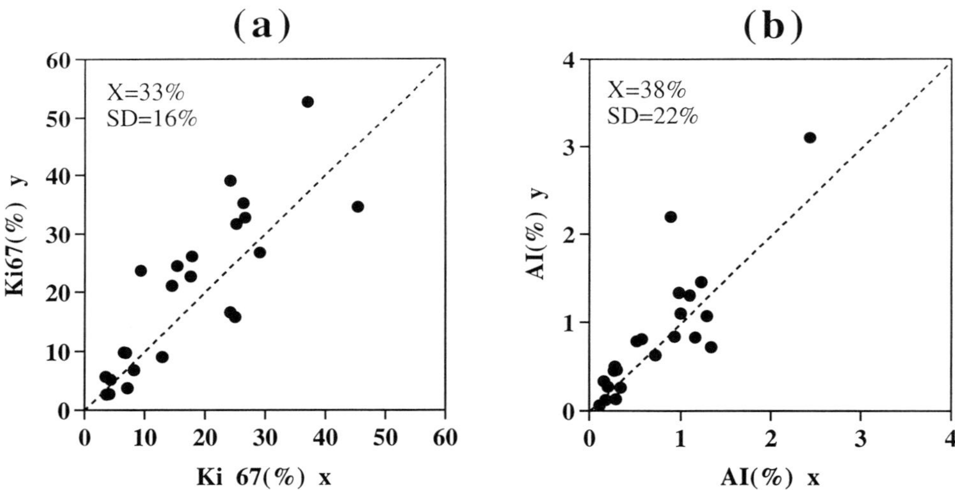

Fig. 1. Intratumoral variability of Ki67 (a) and apoptotic index (AI) (b) as shown by pairs of 14-gauge core-cuts taken immediately after one another from different sites (x and y) of the same breast carcinoma. X = mean difference, SD = standard deviation of the difference. The dashed line is the line of perfect correlation.

Endocrine therapy

Numerous studies of hormonal therapy and breast cancer have established that very few patients with ER-negative disease respond to therapy. These and other data are documented in detail in other chapters of this volume (Miller, Howell, Robertson). We have conducted a small number of studies investigating the changes which occur in what may be considered pivotal biomarkers during tamoxifen therapy.

In a series of 19 patients, nine of whom responded to therapy, ER levels in repeated core-cuts fell from 33.0 ± 17.9% cells staining to 20.5 ± 12.7% and 12.0 ± 16.0% after 1-3 and 4-6 months, respectively [9]. Progesterone receptor (PgR) levels also fell with treatment. Whilst this progressive fall in ER levels with therapy would be consistent with the selection of an ER-negative phenotype, other studies by our group indicate that development of this phenotype is not a significant feature of acquired tamoxifen resistance [10]. These data are similar to those of Robertson et al. [see chapter in this volume].

In the same study all five responding patients in whom paired Ki67 measurements were available showed a decrease in staining (mean pre-treatment: 28.0 ± 8.4%; after 1-3 months, to 9.2 ± 4.8%). There was no consistent change in non-responders (pre-treatment, 32.8 ± 15.8%; after 1-3 months 20.0 ± 10.4%; after 4-6 months 29.2 ± 8.7%).

More recently we have studied changes in hormone receptors and proliferation markers in FNAs taken before and after 14 days' tamoxifen treatment. Importantly, these data confirmed the association of response with decreased Ki67 recorded above: the group of eight patients who eventually responded to treatment showed a significant reduction in Ki67 and there was no significant change in the six non-responders (p = 0.005) [8]. The data have been increased to a total of 22 patients (11 responders, 11 non-responders) and the relationship is maintained (Fig. 2).

These data provide support for early changes in proliferation during hormone therapy being valid intermediate markers of response. This is important given the increasing usage of this parameter in the development and comparison of new drugs [e.g. 11].

Chemotherapy

Our studies of repeat sampling of patients during their treatment with ECF (epirubicin, cisplatin and 5-fluorouracil) indicated for the first time that chemotherapy induces measurable increases in apoptosis in human breast carcinomas within 24 hours of starting therapy. Our initial report showed an overall increase in the percentage of apoptotic cells from a median of 0.47% to 1.02% (p = 0.009) [12]. Ten of the 17 patients showed an increase of >50%, which can be considered significant for individual patients (see above). We have now confirmed that changes of this degree occur in a further series of 22 patients [13]. In

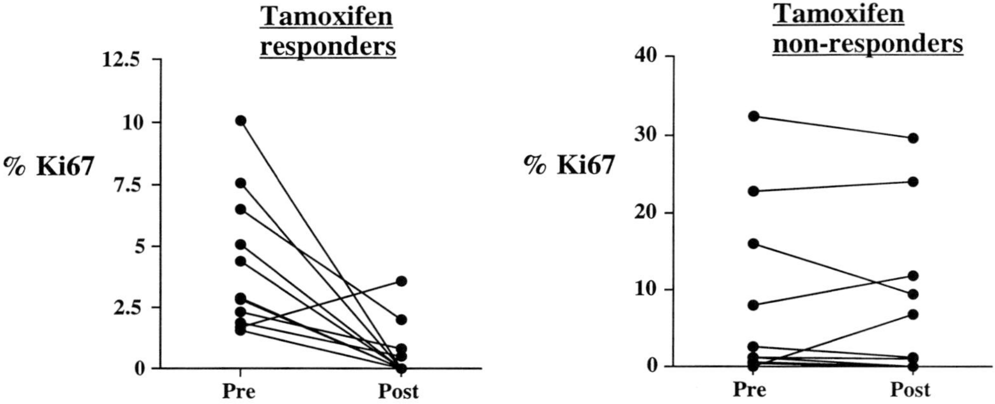

Fig. 2. Change in Ki67 (%) after 14 days of treatment with tamoxifen in 11 responders and 11 non-responders. Measurements were made on cytospins of FNAs.

our first series we reported [12] no significant change in proliferation as measured by Ki67, although there was a trend (median pre-treatment, 19.2%; 24 hours, 15.8%, p = 0.16). However, statistical analysis of a total of 35 patients from the two series revealed a highly significant fall (median pre-treatment, 28.5%; 24 hours, 16.9%, p = 0.009). Only nine of the 35 patients showed a >50% fall, which makes this change after 24 hours less likely to be usable as an index of response than the change in apoptosis. It does, nonetheless, indicate that it may be valuable to study potential determinants of change in proliferation within such samples (e.g. cyclins and cyclin-dependent kinases and their inhibitors).

We also found that the c-erbB2 status of the tumour was significantly related to the change in apoptosis [13]. Nine of the 39 patients (23%) were c-erbB2 positive. In this group the mean increase in apoptotic index at 24 hours (as a percentage of baseline) was 34% compared with 245% in the c-erbB2-negative group (p = 0.02). These data emphasise that the changes in apoptosis and proliferation may themselves be considered appropriate indices of biological response when assessing markers which may be associated with chemoresistance. This point is emphasised by data from our xenograft experiments [14], which showed that marked decreases in proliferation and/or increases in apoptosis can occur without being associated with what would be described as an objective regression in a clinical context (Fig. 3). Whilst such changes may be expected to slow tumour growth, initial rates of apoptosis and proliferation will need to be included into any algorithms to predict actual regression, perhaps in the form of a growth index [14].

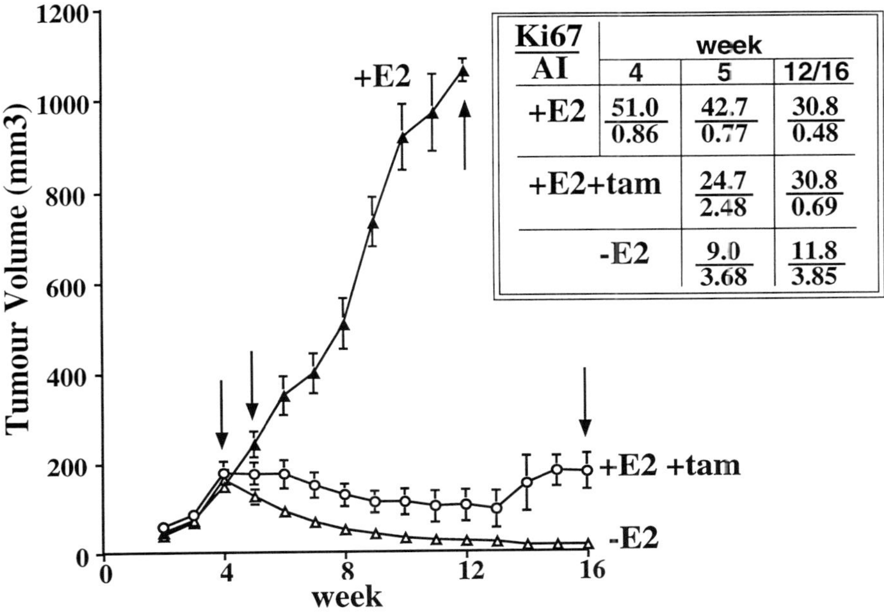

Ki67 / AI	week		
	4	5	12/16
+E2	51.0 / 0.86	42.7 / 0.77	30.8 / 0.48
+E2+tam		24.7 / 2.48	30.8 / 0.69
-E2		9.0 / 3.68	11.8 / 3.85

Fig. 3. Growth curves of MCF7 human breast cancer xenografts grown with oestradiol (E2) support for 4 weeks; then treatment was either continued with E2 alone or tamoxifen treatment was added or E2 was withdrawn. Ki67 (%) and AI (%) were measured at the points shown by the arrows and are shown as Ki67/AI ratios. It is notable that there are substantial changes in both Ki67 and AI after one week of tamoxifen and, although growth ceased, there was no objective regression of tumours.

We have extended our studies of changes in Ki67 with chemotherapy by making measurements after 21 days in patients treated with MM (mitoxantrone, methotrexate) [15]. Eleven of the 12 patients who eventually responded to therapy showed a decrease in Ki67: pre-treatment median levels of 35.2% fell to 5.2% after 21 days, with a mean fall of 68% (percentage of baseline). In contrast, all four of the non-responders showed an increase (Fig. 4). Although the numbers of patients in the non-responders group was very small, these data suggest that change in proliferation after this time is a potential intermediate response indicator, as is argued for treatment above.

Apoptotic index, proliferation (Ki67) and bcl-2 expression have also been measured after three months of ECF in comparison with pre-treatment values. It should be noted that the measurements could not be made in nearly half the patients because there was insufficient residual tumour tissue at operation (c. 20% complete clinical response), leaving 20 patients in whom paired analyses could be made [7]. Median Ki67 levels fell from 8.0% (range: 0.3-41.3%) to 1.3% (0.2-21.9%, p = 0.004) and apoptotic index from 0.59% (0.21-1.8%) to 0.24% (0.10-0.87%, p = 0.004). Thirteen of the 20 patients were positive for bcl-2 pre-

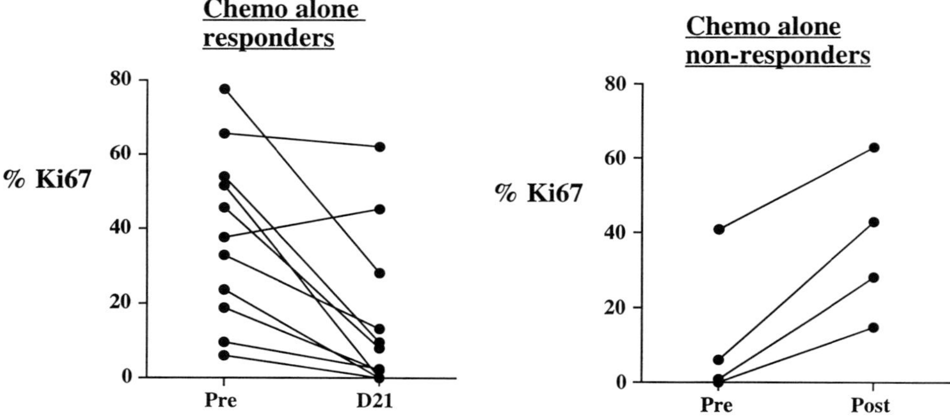

Fig. 4. Change in Ki67 (%) after 21 days of treatment with MM chemotherapy in 12 responders and 4 non-responders. Measurements were made on cytospins of FNAs.

treatment and remained so after treatment; five of the seven patients who were negative pre-treatment were positive after three months' treatment. Overall, the median pre-treatment score of 56% cells positive increased to 80% (p = 0.03).

The change in proliferation and apoptosis is particularly well illustrated by comparison of the scattergrams showing the correlation between apoptotic index and Ki67 pre-treatment and after three months of ECF (Fig. 5) [16]. Prior to

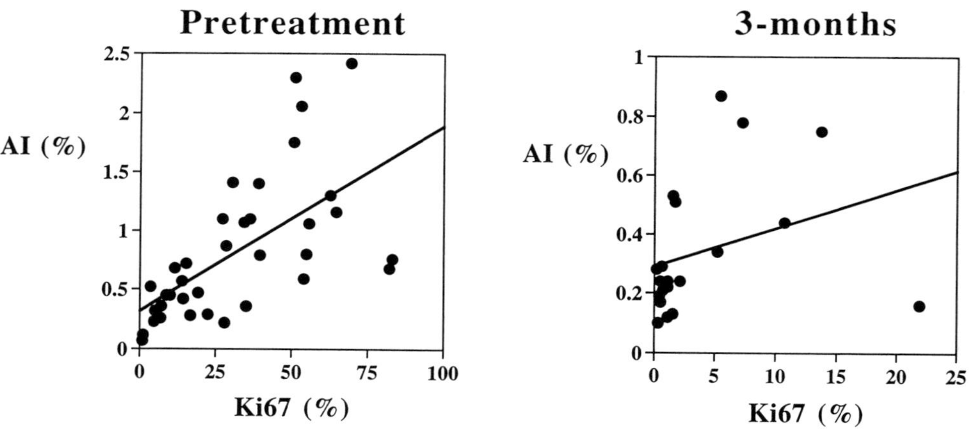

Fig. 5. Relationship between Ki67 and apoptotic index in human breast carcinomas before and three months after the start of chemotherapy. In both cases the relationships were statistically significant: pre-treatment, rho = 0.723, p <0.0001; 3 months, rho = 0.492, p = 0.03. The regression lines are only indicative as the data are not normally distributed.

the therapy there is a strong relationship between the two parameters (rho = 0.723, p <0.0001), which has been reported by others [17]. After treatment, a weaker but still statistically significant relationship persisted (rho = 0.492, p = 0.03), with the majority of the patients having a very low apoptotic and proliferative activity. Thus for those patients who have sufficient tissue for analysis the residual cell population appears to be quiescent or dormant: there is little proliferation but there is also little cell death. The increase in bcl-2 expression is consistent with this protein's anti-apoptotic function, but cannot be necessarily considered as causative of the reduced apoptosis. Further study of the mechanisms which may underlie the phenotype of this residual population should be a priority.

Chemoendocrine therapy

Biological relationships between molecular markers and therapy in breast cancer may be best studied when the treatment is simple (e.g. single agent). However, if the objective of therapy is to achieve maximal downstaging, with the ultimate aim being complete pathological response, then combination therapy is inevitable at present. Recent overview analyses [18,19] have emphasised the additive benefit from combination chemotherapy and tamoxifen. We have therefore conducted clinical studies of chemoendocrine therapy and derived a substantial amount of biological data from one study in particular, in which 300 patients were randomised to either adjuvant or three months neoadjuvant MM plus tamoxifen (MMT). The clinical data are reported in detail elsewhere in this volume [see chapter by Assersohn & Powles].

The relationship between response to MMT and six immunohistochemical markers (ER, PgR, p53, bcl-2, c-erbB2 and Ki67) was examined initially in FNAs taken from between 45 and 80 patients: sample availability and suitability varied between analytes [20]. SPF and ploidy were measured in a further 60 to 71 patients by flow cytometry. The only parameter which shared a significant relationship with clinical response was c-erbB2: 8/14 (57%) positive patients showed a response compared with 29/31 (93%) negative patients, p = 0.007). This relationship has been confirmed in a recent update of the data in whom 100 patients were analysed [21] and by a study of c-erbB2 in the residual tumour of the neoadjuvant patients at surgery [22]. The fact that this oncogene is the only marker of the six to be statistically related to outcome from chemoendocrine therapy may be due to the following: (i) ER, PgR and bcl-2 are markers of good response to endocrine therapy with there being a trend to poor response to chemotherapy; (ii) reverse relationships, i.e. good response to chemotherapy and poor to endocrine therapy, are seen for proliferation (Ki67); (iii) it has become increasingly clear that immunocytochemistry for p53 is unsatisfactory to establish its biological significance [see Lønning et al. in this volume].

We have assessed the change in Ki67 in FNAs taken from 35 patients before and 21 days after starting treatment with MMT [15,23] in analogous studies to

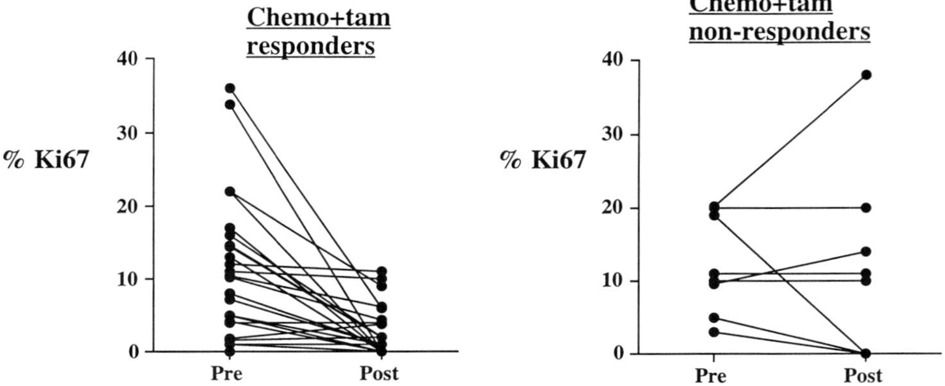

Fig. 6. Change in Ki67 (%) after 21 days of treatment with MMT chemoendocrine therapy in 27 responders and 8 non-responders. Measurements were made on cytospins of FNAs.

those cited above for tamoxifen and MM when applied separately. Again a strong relationship between decrease in proliferation and response was found (Fig. 6). In an earlier smaller study no significant relationship was found between response and change in ER, PgR, p53, bcl-2 or SPF [23].

At the end of three months' chemoendocrine therapy, as with chemotherapy (see above) both Ki67 and apoptotic index were lower than seen in a randomised control group of untreated tumours. In the treated tumours, both Ki67 and AI showed a significant relationship with response (Table 2) [24], with patients who had shown an objective response having significantly lower values than those who had no change or progressive disease. These results are clearly consistent with the observations made above that substantial falls in proliferation occur in responders but not in non-responders to chemoendocrine therapy.

Table 2. Median levels of Ki67 and apoptotic index (AI) in breast carcinomas after three months' treatment with chemoendocrine therapy (MMT) and their relationship with response.

	CR/MRD	PR	NC/PD	p
Ki67 (%)	1.25	2.9	19.6	0.016
n	32	25	12	
AI (%)	0.15	0.28	0.48	0.008
n	23	20	8	

CR, complete response; MRD, minimal residual disease; NC, no change; PD, progressive disease; n = number of patients. Not all samples had sufficient cells for both analyses.

A further finding obtained by comparing samples from patients receiving no presurgical therapy and those receiving three months of MMT was that angiogenesis levels were lower in the pre-treatment group. The median Chalkey score in 90 MMT patients was 5.7 (95% CI 5.3 - 6.0) and in 105 untreated patients 6.3 (95% CI 6.0 - 6.7; p = 0.025). It is not known whether these differences in microvessel density are due to therapy directly causing a reduction in angiogenesis or are secondary to tumour regression [25].

Discussion

Data from the NSABP-B18 study [see review in this volume by Assersohn & Powles] has demonstrated that clinical response to primary chemotherapy is a good indicator of long-term outcome, with pathological complete response being the strongest determinant. Thus, biomarkers that are measured prior to treatment or changes in biomarkers shortly after starting treatment that are strongly predictive of response may themselves be markers of long-term outcome, although this would need to be demonstrated directly.

Our studies have identified a small number of parameters which merit further study in this context. Increases in apoptosis and decreases in proliferation are common factors in response to endocrine therapy and chemotherapy. Relationships with response have yet to be confirmed for apoptosis but are consistent across studies for changes in Ki67 after two to three weeks. The predictive power of these changes needs to be established in larger studies. c-erbB2 status is indicative of a poor response to both chemo and endocrine therapy. Further studies in relation to anthracyclines and taxanes may make this a clinically utilisable observation.

The early changes in proliferation and apoptosis which occur within a day of starting chemotherapy present this as a very valuable scenario for the investigation of the molecular determinants of these changes (e.g. p53, $p21^{cip1}$, bcl-2 family, activation of caspases, cyclins); indeed, certain of these parameters may be revealed as earlier and/or more sensitive markers than proliferation and apoptosis themselves. The application of microarray analyses to clinical samples taken during this period at the time of maximal clinical response may reveal yet more clinically important biological data. Overall it seems clear that molecular and biochemical analyses in association with controlled clinical trials of primary medical therapy will remain one of the most valuable areas of translational research in breast cancer.

Acknowledgements

We would like to acknowledge the contribution made to our studies by Prof. Craig Allred, San Antonio Health Science Center. The work has been supported by grants from the US Army Breast Cancer Command (DAMD 17-97-1-7335), Breast Cancer Research Trust and the NHS R&D Executive.

References

1   Forrest APM, Chetty U, Miller WR et al. A human tumour model. Lancet 1986; ii: 840-2
2   Fernando IN, Powles TJ, Dowsett M et al. Determining factors which predict response to primary medical therapy in breast cancer using a single needle aspirate with immunocytochemical staining and flow cytometry. Virchows Archiv 1995; 426: 155-61
3   Dowsett M, Makris A, Ellis P et al. Oncogene products and other diagnostic markers in human breast cancer patients: Treatment effects and their significance. Ann NY Acad Sci 1996; 784: 403-13. Proceedings of "Biology and biochemistry of normal and cancer cell growth: Propedeutics to cancer management". April 1st-6th 1995, Erice, Sicily
4   Makris A, Allred DC, Powles TJ et al. Cytological evaluation of biological prognostic markers from primary breast carcinomas. Breast Cancer Res Treat 1997; 44: 65-74
5   Ellis PA, Makris A, Burton SA et al. Comparison of MIB-1 proliferation index and S-phase fraction in human breast carcinomas. Br J Cancer 1996; 73: 640-3
6   Dowsett M, Detre S, Ormerod M et al. Analysis and sorting of apoptotic cells from fine needle aspirates of excised human primary breast carcinomas. Cytometry 1998; 32: 291-300
7   Ellis PA, Smith IE, Detre S et al. Reduced apoptosis and proliferation and increased bcl-2 in residual breast cancer following preoperative chemotherapy. Breast Cancer Res Treat 1998; 48: 107-16
8   Makris A, Powles TJ, Allred DC et al. Changes in hormone receptors and proliferation markers in tamoxifen treated breast cancer patients and the relationship with response. Br Cancer Res Treat 1998; 48: 11-20
9   Dowsett M, Johnston, SRD, Detre S et al. Cytological evaluation of biological variables in breast cancer patients undergoing primary medical treatment. In: Motta M, Serio M, eds. Sex hormones and antihormones in endocrine dependent pathology: Basic and clinical aspects. Elsevier, Amsterdam 1994; 329-36
10   Johnston SRD, Saccani-Jotti G, Smith IE et al. Changes in ER, PgR, pS2 expression in tamoxifen resistant human breast cancer. Cancer Res 1995; 55: 3331-8
11   DeFriend DJ, Howell A, Nicolson RI et al. Investigation of a new pure antiestrogen (ICI 182780) in women with primary breast cancer. Cancer Res 1994; 54: 408-14
12   Ellis PA, Smith IE, McCarthy K, Detre S, Salter J, Dowsett M. Preoperative chemotherapy induces apoptosis in early breast cancer (Research letter). Lancet 1997; 349: 849
13   Archer CD, Ellis PA, Dowsett M, Smith IE. C-erbB-2 positivity correlates with poor apoptotic response to chemotherapy in primary breast cancer. Breast Cancer Res Treat 1998; 50: 237
14   Johnston SRD, Boeddinghaus IM, Riddler S et al. Idoxifene antagonises oestradiol-dependent MCF-7 breast cancer xenograft growth through sustained induction of apoptosis. Cancer Res 1999 (submitted)
15   Assersohn L, Powles TJ, Dowsett M, Chang J, Makris A, Trott P. Changes in MIBI expression relate to response in patients receiving primary medical therapy for carcinoma of the breast. Breast Cancer Res Treat 1998; 50: 239
16   Dowsett M, Archer C, Assershon RK et al. Clinical studies of apoptosis and proliferation in breast cancer. Endocrine-Related Cancer 1999 (in press)
17   Lipponen P, Aaltomaa S, Kosma V-M, Syrjanen K. Apoptosis in breast cancer as related to histopathological characteristics and prognosis. Eur J Cancer 1994; 30A: 2068-73
18   Early Breast Cancer Trialists' Collaborative Group. Polychemotherapy for early breast cancer: an overview of randomised trials. Lancet 1998; 352: 930-42
19   Early Breast Cancer Trialists' Collaborative Group. Tamoxifen for early breast cancer: an overview of randomised trials. Lancet 1998; 351: 1451-66
20   Makris A, Powles TJ, Dowsett M et al. Prediction of response to neoadjuvant chemo-endocrine therapy in preliminary breast carcinomas. Clin Cancer Res 1997; 3: 593-600

21 Chang J, Powles TJ, Allred DC et al. Biologic markers predict clinical outcome to chemotherapy for primary operable breast cancer. J Clin Oncol 1999 (submitted)
22 Gregory RK, Powles TJ, Dowsett M, Salter J, Chang JC, Ashley S. Prognostic and predictive relevance of cerbB2 expression in patients in a randomised trial of neo-adjuvant versus adjuvant chemo-endocrine therapy. Ann Oncol 1999 (in press)
23 Makris A, Powles TJ, Allred DC et al. Quantitative changes in cytological molecular markers during primary medical treatment of breast cancer. Breast Cancer Res Treat 1999; 55: 51-9
24 Wu J, Ellis PA, Makris A et al. Differences in ER, Ki67 and Bcl-2 expression in primary human breast cancer before and after treatment with neoadjuvant chemoendocrine therapy. Breast Cancer Res Treat 1996; 41: 240
25 Makris A, Powles TJ, Kokolyris S, Dowsett M, Ashley SE, Harris AL. Reduction in angiogenesis after neoadjuvant chemoendocrine therapy in operable breast cancer. Cancer 1999 (in press)

ESO Scientific Updates, Vol. 4
Primary Medical Therapy for Breast Cancer
A. Howell and M. Dowsett, editors

Primary Medical Therapy: Current Status and Questions which Need to be Answered

Anthony Howell and Mitch Dowsett

The papers presented in this Scientific Update have summarised the current status of primary medical therapy (PMT) for breast cancer. The results of trials of primary chemotherapy (PCT) and primary endocrine therapy (PET) have been reviewed together with a large number of clinical-laboratory studies aimed at improving treatment choices and predicting long-term outcome. It is clear that we have learned a great deal over the past 20 years but, not surprisingly, there remain many unanswered questions. Below we summarise our own estimate of what we know about PMT from the clinical and laboratory viewpoint and highlight the questions we believe need to be answered in order to make progress with this approach to breast cancer treatment.

Primary chemotherapy: what we know

- Most regimens of PCT result in high complete and partial remission rates.
- Response to PCT is a favourable prognostic factor. In some studies only pathological complete responses (pCR) indicate a favourable prognosis.
- Disease-free and overall survival after PCT is not significantly different when the same treatment is given as an adjuvant after surgery.
- Rates of breast conservation are increased after PCT.

Primary chemotherapy: what we need to know

- Can we improve the pCR rates by using newer approaches to chemotherapy (e.g. sequencing of taxanes and anthracyclines or intensifying treatment by increasing dose and reducing treatment intervals)? Will such improvement translate to improved long-term outcome?
- How effective are new chemotherapeutic agents and new combinations of PCT with respect to pCR rates?

- Should additional adjuvant chemotherapy be given after PCT in high-risk disease?

The question of sequencing of taxanes and anthracyclines is being answered by randomised trials of PCT in the USA (NSABP, with taxotere as the taxane) and in Europe (organised from Milan, with taxol as the taxane). These studies will give us information on pCR rates of the sequences and whether they are superior when given before surgery compared with adjuvant use of the same agents. Preliminary information (ASCO, May 1999) indicates high pCR rates for taxanes. The highest pCR rate reported was 30% [1]. This compares favourably with high pCR rates reported previously for platinum containing regimens [2].

Pathological CR appears to be the most important indicator of the effectiveness of PCT and subsequent patient outcome. It is possible that pCRs may be increased by high-dose or "dose dense" therapies. Studies to test this approach are in progress. We might consider only progressing these approaches to randomised studies if they increase pCR rates. Similar arguments might apply to new chemotherapeutic agents and new combinations of drugs.

Primary endocrine therapy: what we know

- High response rates to tamoxifen are seen in patients with ER-positive tumours.

- Response to tamoxifen and possibly other endocrine agents may take many months.

- Higher and more rapid responses may occur with new aromatase inhibitors (see chapter by Miller et al.). These data require confirmation in comparative randomised trials.

- Continuing PET until tumour progression reduces survival and local control compared with primary surgery (see chapter by Howell and Robertson).

Primary endocrine therapy: what we need to know

- Does primary endocrine therapy improve survival?
- Does PET allow more breast conservation surgery? What proportion of responses are pCRs?
- Does achievement of a pCR, CR or PR indicate a good prognosis?
- What is the optimal duration of PET, short or long? If long, how long?
- What is the best agent to use?
- Are combinations of endocrine agents superior to single agents?
- What is the optimal adjuvant therapy after PET?

Although there are a large number of studies concerning PET, they have not been designed to answer the questions listed above. As outlined in the chapter by Howell and Robertson, the reason for this is that PET was seen for many years as a method to avoid surgery in the elderly. The combined results of two randomised trials show that delaying surgery until the time of progression on PET is associated with a moderate survival disadvantage and also results in more examples of uncontrolled local disease.

There is great need to find out the answers to several fundamental questions with respect to PET. We do not know whether PET improves survival since we have no appropriate randomised trials reported or in progress. The optimal studies should compare long (say six months) and short (say two to four weeks) PET compared to untreated controls in patients with ER-positive tumours. All patients would have to have five years of standard adjuvant endocrine therapy. It is possible that PET, which could also be given throughout the surgical period, will result in improved survival. If this was the case we may look back and ask why this approach was not tested appropriately sooner.

Most PET trials were performed using tamoxifen. The Edinburgh group (see chapter by Miller et al.) showed that more rapid responses and increased response rates may be seen using the newer aromatase inhibitors, anastrozole and letrozole. Other new agents which may also be superior to tamoxifen need to be assessed, e.g. the antioestrogens Faslodex, raloxifene, SERM 3 and SCH75050. Ideally there should be a concerted effort to assess all these agents in randomised phase II trials in order to determine which is most active before we embark on phase III trials.

Laboratory studies: what we know

- Oestrogen receptor measurements give high specificity for response to PET but lower sensitivity (see Miller et al.).

- Results concerning the value of markers of proliferation and cell death show that they are inconsistent when measured on the primary tumour before treatment (see Daidone et al.).

- Measurement of markers before and after a period of one to three weeks after the start of PMT may give more precise prediction of response (see Dowsett et al.).

- Mutations in some regions of the TP53 gene and the mdr protein are promising markers of non-responsiveness (see Lønning et al.).

- At present there are no reliable tumour measurements which give accurate prediction of outcome, although several taken together may predict the relapse-free interval (see Daidone et al.).

Laboratory studies: what we need to know

- Are there markers which increase the sensitivity of prediction of endocrine responsiveness?
- Can we derive accurate predictors of chemo-unresponsiveness and pCR?
- Can we identify accurate prognostic markers measured before therapy, perhaps for use in conjunction with initial tumour size and nodal involvement at surgery?
- At present, all the laboratory-based studies are investigational, and – with the exception of ER measurements – none can be advocated for routine use. However, measurements made at two time points (before and after two to four weeks of treatment) appears a promising approach. At present, a limited number of potential markers can be measured. However, with the advent of RT-PCR (see chapter by Magdelénat) and multiple array technology large numbers of markers may be assessed. Although the application of such methods may be regarded as "fishing exercises", their application in carefully followed up large cohorts of patients is, perhaps, the most productive way of improving the laboratory contribution to patient management, which, for all the excellence of the studies performed is, at present, limited.

References

1   Chollet P, Bougnoux P, Amat S et al. Induction chemotherapy in operable breast cancer: high pathological response rate induced by docetaxel. Proc ASCO 1999; 18: 79a
2   Clemons M, Leahy M, Valle J et al. Review of recent trials of chemotherapy for advanced breast cancer: studies excluding taxanes. Eur J Cancer 1997; 33: 2171-82

Subject Index